D1578809

Understanding
Parkinson's Disease

Professor Tony Schapira

*Sponsored by an educational grant
from*

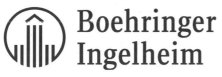

**Boehringer
Ingelheim**

Published by Family Doctor Publications Limited
in association with the British Medical Association

IMPORTANT

This book is intended not as a substitute for personal medical advice but as a supplement to that advice for the patient who wishes to understand more about his or her condition.

Before taking any form of treatment
YOU SHOULD ALWAYS CONSULT YOUR MEDICAL PRACTITIONER.

In particular (without limit) you should note that advances in medical science occur rapidly and some information about drugs and treatment contained in this booklet may very soon be out of date.

Acknowledgements
I am indebted to the many Parkinson's disease patients whom I have seen over the years. Their comments and reflections upon their disease have guided the design of this book. The role of the Parkinson's Disease Society in acting as sponsor, informant and advocate for their members is both recognised and acknowledged. I am indebted to Dr Diane Playford for writing the chapter 'Living with Parkinson's disease'. Her expertise in this area has been invaluable and her chapter will no doubt be of great value to readers. Finally, I thank our Parkinson's disease nurse specialist, Ms Cathy McGee, for reviewing and commenting on the book and for reviewing the role of the nurse specialist.

Dedication
To my wife Laura and my daughter Sarah for their constant understanding and inspiration.

Family Doctor Publications, PO Box 4664, Poole, Dorset BH15 1NN

ISBN: 1 903474 25 6

Contents

About the author

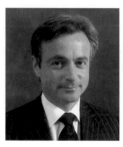

Professor Tony Schapira is Professor of Clinical Neurosciences and a consultant neurologist with considerable experience in treating patients with Parkinson's disease. He has a particular interest in the cause of the disease and in helping to develop new treatments.

Introduction

What is Parkinson's disease?

This book aims to give you an understanding of Parkinson's disease presented in a straightforward and accessible way. If you, or a close friend or relative, has the disease, it will help you deal positively with treatment and daily living. Or you may read it out of general interest or to bring yourself up to date.

Parkinson's disease is one of the most common disorders of the nervous system. It affects muscle movement and many of its symptoms are caused by loss of nerve cells in a very small part of the brain. The main features are tremor, muscle stiffness and slower movements, and these eventually cause the person with the disease to have a characteristic appearance and way of walking.

If you are to have a clear picture of the disease you will need to understand the structure and functions of the brain, and these are explained in the first chapter. The next three chapters give an account of the features of the disease, how it is recognised and what is known about the causes. It was first described in 1817 by Dr James Parkinson, a GP in London. The disease has probably been around for hundreds of years but seems more common now. This would be expected because Parkinson's disease occurs mostly in those over the age of 60 or 70, and nowadays many more people are living beyond that age. Doctors are also now more aware of Parkinson's disease and are able to diagnose it more frequently. Some have suggested that other possible factors, including environmental pollution, might contribute to an increase of the disease (see pages 28–9).

Medical research has identified some of the biochemical causes of the disease and how these affect brain function, causing the typical symptoms. Most importantly, research has led the way to treatment of these symptoms. The treatment of the disease with drugs is described in detail in the chapter starting on page 50.

New drugs introduced in the past 10 years have led to dramatic changes in the control of symptoms and in the outlook for people newly diagnosed with Parkinson's disease. Today, much research is focused on developing treatments that slow or prevent the progression of the disease – and it is likely that such drugs will become available over the next 10 years. As advances are made, some parts of this book will become outdated. We will continually review this and update the book as necessary.

The later chapters in the book discuss the practical aspects of living with Parkinson's disease – which will be helped greatly if you make full use of the support that is available from health professionals such as physiotherapists and specialist nurses. I am particularly indebted to Dr Diane Playford for writing the chapter on 'Living with Parkinson's disease' (page 9).

I dedicate this book to patients with Parkinson's disease, their partners and other family members – they provide an inspiration to others who are faced with less important challenges in life. I also dedicate it to the doctors and scientists who are working towards developing a cure for the disease.

KEY POINTS

■ Parkinson's disease is one of the most common disorders of the nervous system

■ Parkinson's disease occurs mostly in those over the age of 60 or 70

How the brain works

Different parts of the brain have different functions

As the symptoms of Parkinson's disease result from changes in the brain, it helps to understand a little about how your brain works.

Your brain lies inside your skull, and nerves run from it to your eyes and nose, and through the base of your skull into your vertebral column (your spinal cord). Together this makes your central nervous system. Your brain contains millions of nerve cells and also other types of cells that help nerves to function. You have special types of nerve cells in various parts of your brain and they are used for different functions.

The cortex of your brain is the outer layer and forms the indented surface that makes your brain look rather like a walnut! The cortex is divided into several areas and contains a high proportion of nerve cells. Your motor cortex (so called because it controls movement or motion) is towards the front of your brain and is important in voluntary actions – when you want to move your hand or walk it sends signals down bundles

The central nervous system

The brain and spinal cord form the central nervous system. The brain performs many complex functions, for instance it is the source of our consciousness, intelligence and creativity. It also monitors and controls, through the peripheral nervous system, most body processes – ranging from the automatic, such as breathing, to complex voluntary activities, such as riding a bicycle.

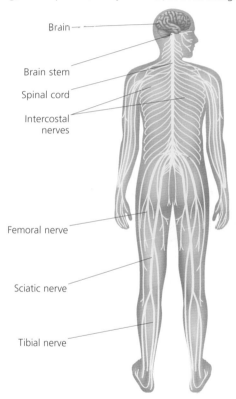

Brain

Brain stem

Spinal cord

Intercostal nerves

Femoral nerve

Sciatic nerve

Tibial nerve

of nerve fibres called the pyramidal tract to the appropriate part of your body.

Your sensory cortex lies a little behind your motor cortex and receives messages about sensations such as touch, heat or vibration.

Sense and movement

Each side of the brain has its own sensory and motor cortices which sense touch and control movement in the opposite side of the body. Movements that involve great complexity or parts of the body that are very sensitive to touch are allocated proportionally larger areas of processing cortex.

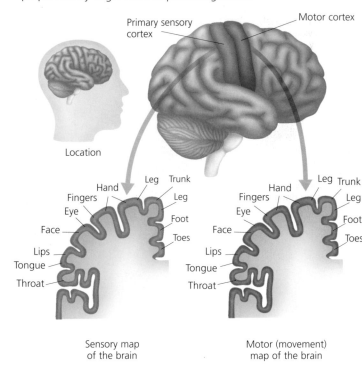

Sensory map
of the brain

Motor (movement)
map of the brain

Your occipital cortex lies at the back of your brain and is involved in sight. It receives signals from your eyes. These signals are 'unscrambled' to form pictures that give us sight.

The cerebellum is separate from the two cerebral hemispheres that form the greater part of your brain. The cerebellum is involved in maintaining balance and

Functions of the brain cortex

Different areas of the brain cortex have specific functions.

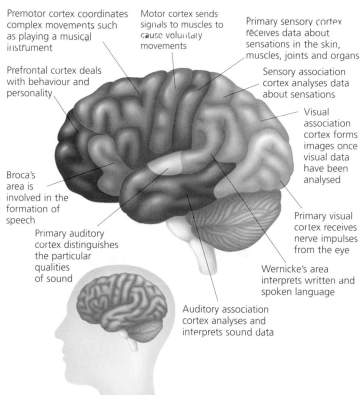

Premotor cortex coordinates complex movements such as playing a musical instrument

Motor cortex sends signals to muscles to cause voluntary movements

Primary sensory cortex receives data about sensations in the skin, muscles, joints and organs

Prefrontal cortex deals with behaviour and personality

Sensory association cortex analyses data about sensations

Visual association cortex forms images once visual data have been analysed

Broca's area is involved in the formation of speech

Primary auditory cortex distinguishes the particular qualities of sound

Primary visual cortex receives nerve impulses from the eye

Wernicke's area interprets written and spoken language

Auditory association cortex analyses and interprets sound data

LOCATION

it enables you to coordinate movements and perform delicate and complex tasks such as playing the piano.

Generally speaking, one side of your brain tends to control movement and sensation over the other side of your body. Some specific functions are located on only one side of your brain – for instance, speech is controlled predominantly by the left side.

The 'cross-over' of brain control

The right and left hemispheres communicate with the muscles and sense organs through nerve bundles that cross from one side of the brain to the other. As a result, the left side of the brain controls the right side of the body and vice versa.

Right hemisphere   **Left hemisphere**

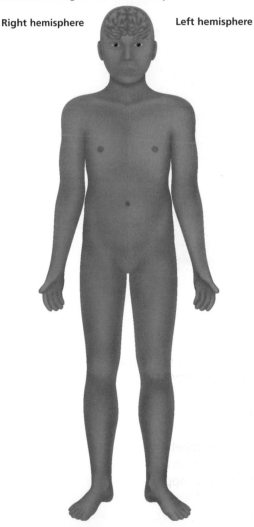

The extrapyramidal system

An area of the brain that is of great importance to Parkinson's disease is the extrapyramidal system (or basal ganglia). This area tunes impulses from other parts of the brain to help control coordinated movements.

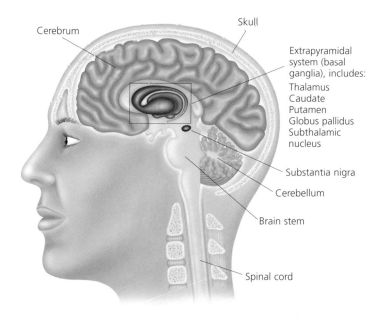

An area that is of great importance to Parkinson's disease is the extrapyramidal system (or basal ganglia), which adds unconscious tuning to the impulses sent down the pyramidal tract. This extrapyramidal tuning is the function of different areas of the brain that appear to work together in organising movement. The names of the parts of the extrapyramidal system are based on their appearance when the brain is examined after death. They include the substantia nigra, the caudate and putamen (which together form the striatum), the thalamus, globus pallidus and subthalamic nucleus.

These areas lie deep within the base of the brain and are connected to the motor cortex. It is in the substantia nigra that there is most loss of nerve cells in Parkinson's disease.

The areas of your brain do not work in isolation – it is the connections between the different nerve cells and areas of the brain that allow it to function in the highly efficient and intricate way that it does.

Nerve cell communications

Nerve cells communicate with each other by two forms of message: one electrical, the other chemical. Nerve cells meet at junctions called synapses. An electrical message passes along a nerve until it reaches the synapse. Here the electrical message is converted into a chemical message by releasing a neurotransmitter from the end of the nerve at the synapse. This neurotransmitter then interacts with receptors on the other side of the synapse. The interaction of the chemical with the receptor is converted into an electrical message that passes along the second nerve. This process is continued so that the message is passed from one nerve to another.

There are different forms of chemical messenger or neurotransmitter in the brain. The cells in the substantia nigra use dopamine as a neurotransmitter. As the number of cells in the substantia nigra falls in Parkinson's disease, so the level of dopamine falls. This affects signals from the substantia nigra to other parts of the brain and interferes with the working of the extrapyramidal system. This results in the symptoms of Parkinson's disease.

How nerve cells transmit signals

Essentially, your brain is like a bundle of telephone wires transmitting and receiving messages within your brain and to and from other parts of your body. Some of the messages are sent by electrical impulses; others depend on the release and transmission of particular chemicals called neurotransmitters.

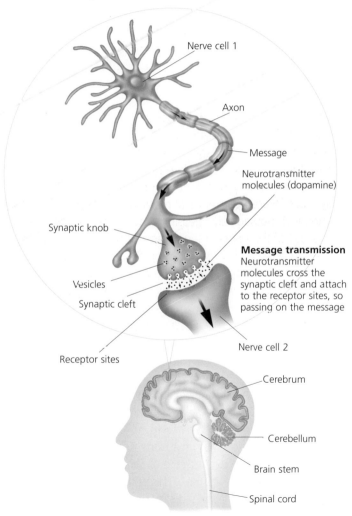

Nerve cell 1

Axon

Message

Neurotransmitter molecules (dopamine)

Synaptic knob

Vesicles

Synaptic cleft

Message transmission
Neurotransmitter molecules cross the synaptic cleft and attach to the receptor sites, so passing on the message

Nerve cell 2

Receptor sites

Cerebrum

Cerebellum

Brain stem

Spinal cord

At the beginning of Parkinson's disease, it is usual for only one side of the brain to be affected or for one side to be affected more than the other. Why one side should be affected before the other remains unexplained.

KEY POINTS

■ An area that appears to be of great importance to Parkinson's disease is the extrapyramidal system located in the 'deep' brain

■ The main symptoms of Parkinson's disease are caused by loss of nerve cells in the substantia nigra

factors is currently the subject of much research – see page 24. Genetic factors are important in explaining the rarer types of the disease that have their onset before the age of 50 (see page 26).

The symptoms of Parkinson's disease

Most frequently, the symptoms of Parkinson's disease develop very gradually over a period of years rather than months. The person affected may be unaware that he or she has symptoms of the disease. The features are often noticed first by a friend or relative who may suggest that the person is 'slowing down' or has a tremor – which the patient had not noticed. Only after the disease has been diagnosed may the patient and the family look back with the benefit of

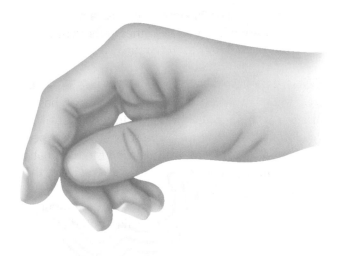

Shaking of one or both hands is the most common early symptom of Parkinson's disease.

hindsight and realise that symptoms (though mild and causing no disability) had been present for a long time.

These first mild symptoms vary, but usually the person gradually develops a collection of features that are characteristic of Parkinson's disease. Not all patients have all symptoms. It is the collection of features together that allows the diagnosis to be made, although it may be suspected earlier by a relative or by the general practitioner. In most cases the GP will refer the person with the disease to a specialist for a definite diagnosis and advice on management.

The following covers some of the more frequent features of the disease.

Slowness

Patients, or their relatives, notice that they tire quickly and are slowing down. This may involve their walking or dexterity. They may feel themselves to be clumsy, especially when trying to do fiddly tasks with their hands such as doing up and undoing buttons. Certain 'automatic' movements become slower. For instance, a patient may blink or swallow less frequently. If swallowing becomes a lot less as the disease progresses, saliva can collect in the mouth and sometimes dribble out of the side of the mouth. The patient's face may seem less mobile and facial movements less spontaneous. At later stages of the disease, if facial movements are very reduced, the person's face can appear 'mask-like'. You may hear your doctors talking about bradykinesia – by which they mean a lack of movement while sitting or standing, that is no crossing or uncrossing of the legs or movement of the arms and hands.

Stiffness

Patients find that they have increasing stiffness, particularly in their arms and legs. This can cause problems in getting dressed. The stiffness is sometimes associated with pain, and many people with Parkinson's disease go to their family doctor with complaints that suggest a 'frozen shoulder'. This is because the muscles around the shoulder and upper limb become stiffer and the pain produced is interpreted as a joint problem. As the stiffness and slowness progress throughout the course of the disease, they combine to affect the person's walking and other tasks (see below).

Tremor

Typically, tremor begins in a hand or foot. It is usually a fine tremor with a movement of a fraction of an inch (five millimetres or less) repeated about three to five times a second. In the hand, it is the thumb, index and middle fingers that are most often affected. The movement can look as if the person is rolling a small ball or 'pill' between the thumb and first two fingers. This has led to the term 'pill-rolling tremor'. The forearm may also be affected with a rotational movement of the hand.

The tremor is typically present at rest and disappears when the person goes to pick something up, although this is not always the case. It is made worse by stress, anxiety or excitement.

Patients can voluntarily suppress the tremor for a short time but this requires concentration and the tremor will return when the attention is switched to something else. The tremor usually disappears during sleep.

Postural instability

As the disease progresses, patients can feel unsteady and may suffer falls. This happens when the disease affects the reflexes that in healthy people allow quick recovery from a trip or stumble. In people with Parkinson's disease the stiffness and slowness make it difficult to correct any imbalance.

Diagnosis and progress

At first these main symptoms of Parkinson's disease (slowness, stiffness, tremor and balance problems) usually affect one side of the body only. As the disease progresses, the other side may become affected. The appearance of the symptoms on one side reflects the loss of nerve cells (neurons) in the substantia nigra on the other side of the brain.

As the symptoms progress, they may affect various activities of daily life. Handwriting typically changes to become smaller (micrographia) and more arduous. Also the tremor, if present in the dominant (writing) hand, may be seen in an individual's script. The loss of dexterity may make it difficult to tie shoelaces and ties or sew. Speech can become softer.

Walking can become affected. Early in the disease, the arm on the affected side does not swing normally

Symptoms of Parkinson's disease

- Slowness
- Stiffness
- Tremor
- Postural instability

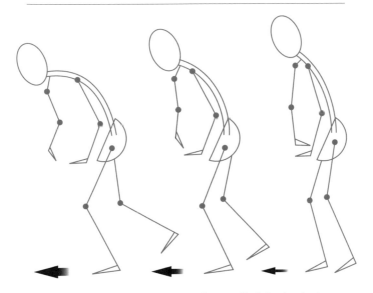

A walk may break into a run. This is called 'festination'.

when the person walks. As the condition progresses, the person may walk with small steps and may become stooped. This adds to the difficulty of balance as it throws the centre of gravity a little forward of the toes and creates an unstable position. The slow, small steps (festinant gait) become more rapid as 'they try to catch up' with their centre of gravity, and a walk may break into a run. After a series of short steps the person may find that the feet have become apparently stuck to the ground, an event known as 'freezing'.

Tremor, slowness and stiffness are the major symptoms, but from the earliest stages people with Parkinson's disease may be troubled by other, so-called minor symptoms. These include constipation, a need to pass urine more frequently and a greasy skin. Some patients are troubled by depression and confusion, symptoms that are often the result of problems with other neurotransmitters (see below).

The rate at which Parkinson's disease will progress varies from one individual to another. Generally speaking, those who present predominantly with tremor do well with slow progression and only mild-to-moderate stiffness or slowness. Young-onset patients tend to progress a little more rapidly at first, but this often tends to stabilise after about 5 to 10 years. Later-onset patients tend to progress slowly over 10 years or so. More advanced disease can become complicated by motor (movement) fluctuations such as dyskinesias (see page 56) or wearing off of the effects of drugs (see pages 54–5).

Outlook

Modern medical management of Parkinson's disease has resulted in substantial improvement in patients' long-term quality of life. Indeed, the vast majority of patients can now look forward to a normal life span.

Disease progression is a reflection of the continuing loss of dopamine-producing neurons in the substantia nigra, and the emergence of nerve cell loss in other areas of the brain that do not involve dopamine. The latter lead to symptoms that are not responsive to drugs that have the same effect as dopamine (dopaminergic drugs) such as levodopa or dopamine agonists. Failure to modify the course of Parkinson's disease is a major limitation of current treatment and is the basis for a considerable research effort to discover neuroprotective drugs.

KEY POINTS

- The chance of a person developing Parkinson's disease in their lifetime is estimated as 1 in 40 to 1 in 50

- The disease is most common after 50 years of age, although it may occur earlier

- The symptoms of Parkinson's disease are slowness, stiffness, tremor and postural instability

The underlying causes of Parkinson's disease

The cause of the symptoms of Parkinson's disease

The symptoms of Parkinson's disease are mainly the result of the loss of cells containing or producing dopamine in the substantia nigra. This affects the working of the extrapyramidal system and causes the typical features of stiffness, rigidity and tremor. These symptoms respond to treatment that helps replace the lost dopamine.

However, the dopamine cells of the substantia nigra are not the only ones to be affected in Parkinson's disease. Some nerve cells, using chemicals known as acetylcholine and 5-hydroxytryptamine (5HT) as neurotransmitters, are also affected in other parts of the brain. The loss of these cells may produce features such as certain types of postural instability (in addition to the problems caused by lack of dopamine), depression and confusion. Clearly, such symptoms will not respond to medication aimed at improving the dopamine system.

Lewy bodies

Microscopic examination of the substantia nigra of a patient with Parkinson's disease shows a loss of dopamine cells. This can be done only after death, from whatever cause, and only with consent. The examination also shows the presence of protein structures called Lewy bodies in some of the surviving nerve cells.

Lewy bodies are made up of a mixture of proteins, including ubiquitin and alpha-synuclein (see 'Genetic factors' below). They can often be seen in other parts of the brain in Parkinson's disease and in some other neurological disorders including a type of dementia. We don't yet know the significance of Lewy bodies in Parkinson's disease.

What causes the loss of the dopamine cells in the substantia nigra?

Over the last few years it has become clear that there is not just one cause of Parkinson's disease but several. Attention is now focused on the role that genetic causes may play in Parkinson's disease, what environmental influences may produce the disorder, and how genetic and environmental factors may work together to cause the disease.

Genetic factors

The genetic contribution to the cause of Parkinson's disease is very complicated, but it has become clear that some genes are involved in certain inherited forms of the disease. Most cases of the disease do not, however, show a clear genetic factor.

Lewy bodies

Microscopic examination of the substantia nigra of a patient with Parkinson's disease shows a loss of dopamine cells and the presence of protein structures called Lewy bodies in some of the surviving nerve cells.

Microscope section of a nerve cell from the substantia nigra

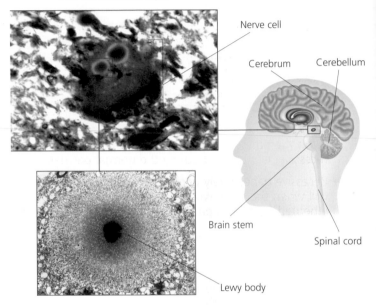

Nerve cell

Cerebrum

Cerebellum

Brain stem

Spinal cord

Lewy body

Electron micrograph of a Lewy body

An individual's genetic material is found in each cell of the body. Most is in the DNA of the chromosomes inside each cell nucleus. A separate and much smaller source of genetic information is in the DNA of mitochondria. Mitochondria are small subsections of a cell that are responsible for producing energy, and damage to the mitochondria plays a part in causing Parkinson's disease.

Genes

- The genes in your body are made up of 30,000 pairs, one of each pair coming from each parent.

- Many of the pairs of genes are identical in structure and action, but some genes have variations (mutations).

- Mutant genes may produce slightly different actions. Geneticists classify mutant genes into two categories: dominant and recessive.

- If one of a pair of genes is mutant and is strong or dominant, it blocks out the activity of the normal gene in the pair and produces an abnormal protein or function.

- If, on the other hand, a mutant gene is weak or recessive, it is blocked out by the normal partner.

- Recessive genes rarely become active and only will when the same type of recessive gene is inherited from both parents.

The DNA from chromosomes is passed from both parents to each offspring, but mitochondrial DNA is passed only from a mother to her children. Each gene is a length of DNA of specific composition. Genes produce proteins, which are the basis for all cells and functions in the body. It is your genes that determine features that vary from one family to another such as hair or eye colour.

Strong genes lead to what is called autosomal dominant inheritance and weak, recessive genes lead to autosomal recessive inheritance. If one parent has an autosomal dominant gene that causes a disease, the gene will be passed on to half of his or her children, so that on average each child will have a 50 per cent chance of being affected. If both parents carry a single weak gene, each child has only a one in four chance of inheriting the mutant gene from both parents and so of having the disease.

The first identified gene mutation

The first gene to be identified as causing Parkinson's disease was found in 1997 in a large American–Italian family and four Greek families. The gene that produces the protein called alpha-synuclein was found to be different (mutated) in these families. It is a strong gene and so the families showed autosomal dominant inheritance of Parkinson's disease.

The gene produces early onset Parkinson's disease, with most affected individuals developing symptoms in their early 40s. The rate of progression is rapid, most dying within 10 years. Mutations in the alpha-synuclein gene are rare. Nevertheless these mutations may prove to be important because scientists are now studying how the alpha-synuclein protein affects the loss of cells in the substantia nigra – and this may provide clues to understanding the more common types of Parkinson's disease.

The second identified gene mutation

The second gene found to cause Parkinson's disease was discovered in a group of Japanese patients who developed the disease as adolescents. The mutation was in a weak (autosomal recessive) gene for a protein called parkin. Mutations in this gene have since been identified in a substantial proportion of young-onset patients in the rest of the world, particularly those whose clinical features appear before the age of 30.

However, parkin mutations have also been identified in patients who developed the disease in their 50s. Interestingly, some patients with only one mutated parkin gene have been described.

Thus, parkin mutations appear to be more common than alpha-synuclein mutations as a cause of Parkinson's disease. Parkin mutations can cause all the major clinical features of Parkinson's disease, often with some unusual features – the Japanese patients showed significant improvement with sleep. It has been possible to examine some brains of patients with parkin mutations and so far no Lewy bodies have been found.

The third identified gene mutation

A third mutation causing Parkinson's disease was found in a single family in the gene that produces a protein called UCH-L1. Parkin and UCH-L1 proteins appear to be involved in the disposal of proteins within nerve cells. So there is now great interest in the way in which proteins are removed when no longer needed in nerve cells, particularly in Parkinson's disease.

Recently identitied gene mutations

Over the past two years mutations in other proteins, for example, DJ-1, Pink-1 and LRRK2, have been described and several others await characterisation.

Separate from the specific gene mutations described above, there appears to be a slightly increased risk of Parkinson's disease developing in a first-degree relative (parent/child/brother/sister) of a patient. This risk is further increased if there are two or more relatives affected. This occurs only in the very few families with strong, dominantly inherited Parkinson's disease, for example, alpha-synuclein mutations, where a gene for the disease can be seen to pass through regularly from one generation to another.

Environmental factors

As there is no clear family history for most Parkinson's disease patients, it is assumed that genes do not play a major role in most patients. So attention has focused on environmental factors that may influence the onset of the disorder.

However, despite numerous studies around the world, no clear environmental influence has been demonstrated as the cause of Parkinson's disease. There are some relatively weak influences that appear to increase slightly the risk of the disorder – such as drinking well water, proximity to wood mills or the use by agricultural workers of pesticides or herbicides – but such factors can contribute to only a very small minority of cases.

Some important clues to the cause of Parkinson's disease came from an unusual 'environmental agent'. In the early 1980s, an unemployed biochemist in California decided to produce a heroin-like drug that he could sell on the streets to addicts. Unfortunately, his chemistry was a little sloppy and his batches were contaminated with a compound called methylphenyl-tetrahydropyridine (MPTP). Some unfortunate addicts who used this as a heroin substitute and injected it into their veins developed Parkinson's disease within one to two weeks.

It was found that MPTP is converted into another compound, MPP+, in the brain, which is then actively absorbed by nerve cells that use dopamine. It goes into the mitochondria and affects the production of energy in the cell. It also causes the production of free radicals (see below), which damage various parts of a cell. So MPP+ is a very potent toxin.

Although it is estimated that about 200 to 400 individuals were exposed to MPTP, only about 10 actually developed Parkinson's disease. This might simply reflect the amount of drug each person took, but it may indicate that some people have a genetic predisposition to the effects of compounds such as MPTP. This has supported the suggestion that some patients with Parkinson's disease may have their illness as a result of a genetic susceptibility as well as exposure to a specific environmental agent.

The importance of studying the brain

All the research into the causes and pathogenesis (the origin and process by which a disease develops) of Parkinson's disease has an important purpose. It will provide an understanding of the likely causes of the illness and the mechanism by which they produce cell loss. This will help to develop treatments that can slow down or prevent the disease. Research in this area is already bearing fruit and several new drugs are currently being tested to see whether they can indeed alter the course of Parkinson's disease and improve the outlook for patients. This is covered in more detail under 'Drugs used in the treatment of Parkinson's disease' (page 50).

The study of the pathogenesis of Parkinson's disease is an investigation into the biochemical abnormalities in the brain induced by genetic causes, environmental factors or both. So far we have some pieces of the puzzle and these are described below. Numerous biochemical abnormalities have been discovered since the MPTP model described above.

Iron deposits

One change identified in the substantia nigra of Parkinson's disease patients is an increase in the deposition of iron. It is probably not a primary cause of Parkinson's disease – increased iron levels are often seen in damaged tissues. Nevertheless, if iron is present in high concentrations and also in a free reactive form (in which it enters easily into chemical reactions with other cell constituents) it can significantly increase the production of damaging free radicals (small, highly active atoms which react with fats and proteins within the cell and so change both their structure and function). So, although the iron may not be a prime event in the cause of Parkinson's disease, it may contribute to brain cell damage.

Energy pathway

MPP+ is concentrated within mitochondria and, once inside, inhibits the action of an enzyme called complex I. This is the first part of a pathway that supplies energy to the cell. The inhibition of the enzyme complex I is, therefore, likely to lead to nerve cell death. Brains have been examined after consent from Parkinson's disease patients who have died from whatever cause, and there was a significant lack of complex I activity in the substantia nigra. This has led to the study of the role of mitochondrial abnormalities in causing Parkinson's disease. Some studies have shown that complex I activity is also low in some tissues such as platelets or muscle. It is possible that this could be used to identify the presence of disease before symptoms develop.

Free radicals

MPP+ is also associated with increased free radical production, which plays a part in the effect of MPTP in inducing Parkinson's disease. The link between free radicals and Parkinson's disease has been strengthened by the identification of increased oxidative stress and damage to cells in the brains of people with Parkinson's disease.

Mitochondria produce most of the free radicals found in a cell. Their numbers are normally carefully controlled and do not damage the cell. However, if a mitochondrion is not working properly it may produce more free radicals. These can damage other mitochondria, which can then leak free radicals into the cell and cause further damage. So the mitochondrial damage and free radical generation in a brain with Parkinson's disease can be both self-perpetuating and self-amplifying.

Calcium

Calcium is critically important to the normal functioning of a cell, and its metabolism and transport in and out of a cell are carefully controlled. There is some evidence for abnormal calcium handling in Parkinson's disease brain cells. This may be as a result of damaged mitochondria, because they are one of the most important sites for calcium accumulation.

Inflammation

Brains from patients with Parkinson's disease show some evidence of inflammation in the substantia nigra. This change has also been seen in other degenerative diseases of the nervous system and is not specific for Parkinson's disease. It is unlikely to be a prime event in the disorder – it's probably a reaction to the abnormalities in the substantia nigra. However, as with increased iron levels, inflammation may contribute to cell damage.

Smoking and caffeine

Some environmental factors have been investigated because they appear to reduce the risk of Parkinson's disease. One of these is smoking. Many studies have shown that Parkinson's disease occurs less often in people who smoke than in non-smokers. We don't yet know how smoking does this. It may be that tobacco smoke contains some protective chemicals, or it may be something in the make-up of smokers themselves. Scientists do not, however, recommend taking up smoking because of its many clearly proven dangers. Another factor is caffeine; again a high intake may reduce the risk of Parkinson's disease but much more research needs to be done.

Biochemical abnormalities

This chapter has already outlined the effects of some biochemical changes in causing Parkinson's disease. Several abnormalities have been identified, particularly in the substantia nigra. The three most consistent changes are evidence for:

- free radical damage
- mitochondrial dysfunction
- inflammation.

Evidence is also emerging that there may be a mechanism of damage termed 'excitotoxicity'.

Free radical damage

Free radicals are atomic (very small) structures that can interact with substances inside the cell to change their structure and therefore alter their function. Free radicals are produced by a variety of means and have a number of purposes – not all bad. Free radicals, for example, are important in fighting infection; certain types of white blood cells kill bacteria by producing free radicals. Generally speaking, however, free radicals are harmful.

The most common type of free radical is produced from oxygen (the superoxide ion). Most of the oxygen radicals produced by a cell are produced in mitochondria as a natural byproduct of the energy-producing pathway. Under normal circumstances, the oxygen radicals are contained within mitochondria but, as suggested above, if mitochondria begin to malfunction, the free radicals leak out and can damage the cell. Other types of free radicals involving free radical-generating molecules include hydrogen peroxide, the hydroxyl ion and nitric oxide.

Free radicals are produced in greater concentration when there is iron present in an abundant and freely reactive form. Free radical damage probably also accumulates as a natural process of ageing, and may even be part of the reason why animals age.

There are numerous defence systems in the body to prevent damage from free radicals. These include enzymes that can turn free radicals into harmless molecules. Also certain vitamins – for example, vitamin E – have a role to play in preventing free radical damage.

There are a number of biochemical changes in the substantia nigra of people with Parkinson's disease that indicate that there is an excess of free radical production in this area, and there is also damage to cells from the free radicals. Such free radical damage has also been seen in tissues in other disorders, including rheumatoid arthritis, and other neurodegenerative disorders such as Alzheimer's disease and Huntington's disease. Thus, free radical damage is not specific for Parkinson's disease.

Mitochondrial dysfunction

As mentioned above, mitochondria have a critical role to play in producing energy for the metabolism of the cell. In addition, it has recently been discovered that mitochondria have an important role in determining when a cell dies, signalled by a decline in their function.

Based on the clues provided by MPTP toxicity, mitochondrial function was investigated in the substantia nigra of patients with Parkinson's disease who had died. It showed a specific deficiency of complex I (energy-synthesising enzyme). This not only established a direct link between Parkinson's disease and MPTP toxicity, but also suggested some possible explanation for why there was free radical damage in the Parkinson's disease brain – namely the loss of normal mitochondrial function.

Mitochondrial abnormalities have also been identified in the blood of a proportion of patients with Parkinson's disease, and some research workers have also found abnormal mitochondrial function in the muscles of some patients. These findings suggest that mitochondrial dysfunction may not be restricted to the brain of people with Parkinson's disease. If this is true and there is widespread mitochondrial dysfunction in Parkinson's disease, it implies that there is an inherited or environmental toxic effect causing it.

As mentioned earlier, mitochondria have their own DNA and this is passed from mothers to all offspring. So if mitochondrial DNA plays a major role in the inheritance of Parkinson's disease, there may be an excess of what is called maternal inheritance, in which a disorder is inherited from the mother but not the father. However, while some research has shown this to be the case, some has found no difference between inheritance from mothers or from fathers. Nevertheless, occasionally mitochondrial DNA mutations have been associated with patients who have developed Parkinson's disease, suggesting that maternal inheritance may sometimes explain the transmission of the disease.

The discovery of complex I deficiency in Parkinson's disease led to some work on a common herbicide called rotenone. Rotenone is a strong and specific inhibitor of mitochondrial complex I, and it was suggested that, if complex I deficiency is important in Parkinson's disease, rotenone may be able to mimic this disorder in an animal experiment.

Indeed, this was demonstrated in rats where slow infusion of rotenone over a period of about a month led to abnormalities in the brain that closely mimicked those found in Parkinson's disease patients. These experiments confirmed the importance of mitochondrial abnormalities in Parkinson's disease and intriguingly raised the possibility that some herbicides or pesticides may be involved in causing it. However, studies looking at the frequency with which exposure to herbicides and pesticides was documented in Parkinson's disease patients before the onset of the disease have not identified any clear role for these chemicals in most such patients.

It is likely that there are multiple causes of Parkinson's disease, and free radical damage and mitochondrial abnormality may only be important in some cases. There may be causes of Parkinson's disease that do not involve either of these processes.

Cross-section of a typical human cell

Cells are the microscopic, basic structural and functional units of all living organisms.

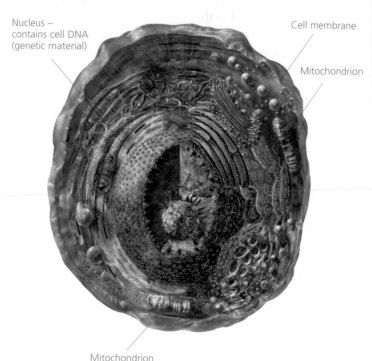

Nucleus – contains cell DNA (genetic material)

Cell membrane

Mitochondrion

Mitochondrion

Inflammation

Inflammation is basically a reaction of the body's defence system to combat some invading organism or, alternatively, to react against abnormal tissue within the body. Blood flow is increased in the inflamed region, bringing in more defensive white blood cells. Inflammation is most commonly seen in infections but inflammatory cells have also been found in the brains of people with certain neurodegenerative disorders.

It is more likely than not that the inflammatory cells present in the substantia nigra of people with Parkinson's disease represent a 'reaction' to the abnormalities found in that area of the brain rather than being a primary cause of the disease. Nevertheless, the inflammatory changes that occur may contribute to nerve cell damage, and combating the inflammation may help to slow down or prevent development of the disorder. There are some new results suggesting that people who take anti-inflammatory tablets, such as those used for arthritis, may be at lower risk of developing Parkinson's disease.

Excitotoxicity

Excitotoxic cell damage refers to damage that may be induced by activation of nerve cells by glutamate. Glutamate is a naturally occurring chemical in the brain which is used as a messenger to relay chemical information between cells. However, activation of nerve cells with glutamate can also initiate a sequence of events that can eventually cause damage to the cell.

This cellular damage is caused by the free radical nitric oxide which is produced within the cell after the glutamate has activated glutamate receptors on the cell surface – the process of excitotoxicity.

Excitotoxicity may play a role in motor neuron disease and Huntington's disease, and evidence for this type of damage has also been found in the nerve cells of patients with Parkinson's disease. Individuals cannot control the amount of glutamate in their brains, and there is no relationship between this and any dietary source.

KEY POINTS

■ Genes have been identified that cause inherited forms of Parkinson's disease

■ No environmental contribution to the cause of Parkinson's disease has yet been clearly defined

■ Free radical damage and mitochondrial dysfunction are important in Parkinson's disease

The diagnosis of Parkinson's disease

The importance of symptoms

As previously described under symptoms (see page 18), the characteristics of Parkinson's disease include slowness, stiffness and tremor. From this, it would seem that the diagnosis of Parkinson's disease is straightforward – but this is not so.

There is no test for the disease, so a diagnosis has to be made from the pattern of symptoms. As the disease develops gradually, it is hard for a doctor to be sure of the diagnosis until enough symptoms are present. Also, many patients do not have all the symptoms, and sometimes the changes are only subtle in the early stages. Furthermore there are a number of disorders that have symptoms similar to Parkinson's disease. If doubt remains, it is best that the doctor should monitor the patient rather than diagnose Parkinson's disease – once a diagnosis is made it can't be reversed without distress.

Many older people do not seek a diagnosis for a number of years because they dismiss the features of

Parkinson's disease as part of the process of ageing. Sadly, such patients suffer their symptoms unnecessarily for several years when they could have benefited from treatment and an improved quality of life.

Although there are no specific tests for Parkinson's disease, certain scans can provide supporting evidence for a clinical diagnosis of Parkinson's disease by measuring the ability of the brain to produce dopamine (see figure on page 41). Such scans use processes called positron emission tomography (PET) or single photon emission computed tomography (SPECT).

Fluorodopa PET scans measure the ability of the brain to produce dopamine and thus reflect the function of the dopamine-containing neurons. These types of scan are not, however, used as a standard diagnostic test for Parkinson's disease. SPECT measures the density of the dopamine transporter – a protein on nerve terminals – and therefore is an indication of the number of surviving dopaminergic neurons.

How the diagnosis is made

When you first go to your doctor with symptoms that might raise the possibility of Parkinson's disease, you will usually be asked numerous detailed questions. These include: the duration of the symptoms, the rate of progression, any other additional symptoms that might suggest an alternative diagnosis, whether there is any family history of Parkinson's disease and, most importantly, whether certain types of medication have been taken (see under 'Disorders that mimic Parkinson's disease', page 44).

The doctor will then examine you. He or she will carefully observe whether there is any tremor at rest, note how you walk and whether or not your arms

SPECT scan

Single photon emission computed tomography (SPECT). A radionuclide is introduced into the body which is taken up by the dopamine transporters in the nerve cells of the brain. The SPECT scan detects the emissions and so builds up a picture that indicates the number of surviving dopaminergic neurons.

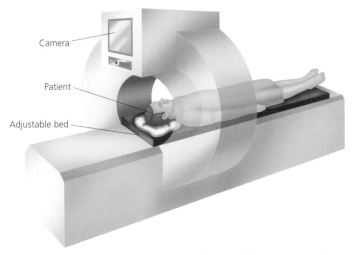

The images, produced over a 48-month period for a representative patient, show the progressive loss of dopamine transporter

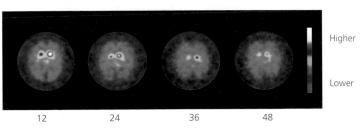

swing freely, whether your steps are normal and how easily you turn without losing balance. If your GP thinks that it is likely that you have Parkinson's disease he or she will probably refer you to a specialist for

Specialist examination

The doctor will carefully observe whether there is any tremor at rest, note how you walk and whether or not your arms swing freely, whether your steps are normal and how easily you turn without losing balance.

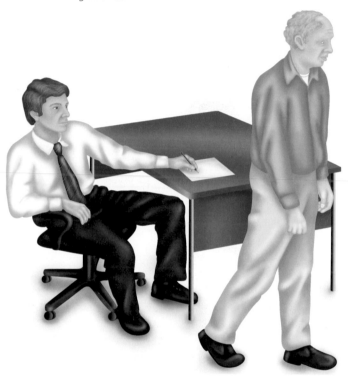

assessment. It is a good idea to ask for a referral to a specialist even if your GP does not suggest it. A specialist such as a neurologist or geriatrician with a special interest in Parkinson's disease is the best person for an accurate diagnosis and for the best treatment.

More detailed neurological examination will include assessment of your speech and eye movements, and a detailed assessment of your limbs, how freely they move,

Computed tomography

Computed tomography (CT) fires X-rays through the brain at different angles. The X-rays are picked up by receivers and the information analysed by a computer to create a picture of the brain.

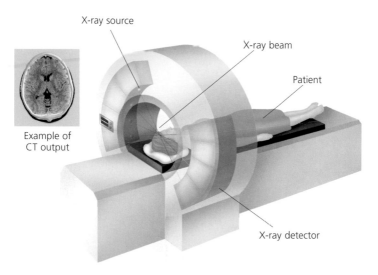

X-ray source

X-ray beam

Patient

Example of CT output

X-ray detector

their strength, your reflexes and, of course, sensation. Important questions are also often asked about control of bladder and bowels. Bladder dysfunction can arise in certain diseases that may mimic Parkinson's disease. Constipation is common among Parkinson's disease patients.

Some tests, such as examination of the blood or urine, may be taken to check for other disorders (see below) that have some symptoms similar to Parkinson's disease. Sometimes you may have an eye examination to exclude other rarer conditions that are similar to Parkinson's disease. Some doctors routinely refer patients for scans by computed tomography (CT) or magnetic resonance imaging (MRI), which can help

Magnetic resonance imaging (MRI)

Magnetic resonance imaging (MRI) uses powerful magnets to align the atoms in the part of the body being studied. Radiowave pulses break the alignment causing signals to be emitted from the atoms. These signals can be measured and a detailed image built up of the tissues and organs.

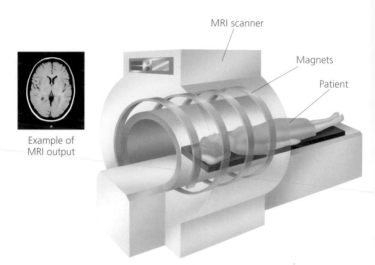

MRI scanner

Magnets

Patient

Example of
MRI output

exclude other diagnoses. Others believe that this is unnecessary if the diagnosis of Parkinson's disease is straightforward.

Disorders that mimic Parkinson's disease
Multiple system atrophy

There is a variety of nervous system disorders grouped under the term 'multiple system atrophy'. These disorders involve malfunction of several parts of the brain including the substantia nigra. The symptoms mimic those of Parkinson's disease but there are usually additional features such as slurring of speech, abnormal movements of the eyes, unsteadiness and changes in the reflexes.

Also, bladder function may be affected because of involvement of nerves to the centres of bladder control. Multiple system atrophy is diagnosed on clinical signs and there is no specific test to distinguish it absolutely from Parkinson's disease. It responds poorly to dopaminergic drugs.

Progressive supranuclear palsy

Progressive supranuclear palsy is another type of disorder that can mimic Parkinson's disease. It is characterised by abnormal eye movements as well as stiffness of the whole body and not just the limbs. Treatment is mainly supportive.

Postencephalitic parkinsonism

Viral infections of the brain can occasionally cause Parkinson's disease. There was an outbreak of postencephalitic parkinsonism at the beginning of the twentieth century. Occasional new cases are still seen, although they are rare. There are some features that distinguish it from normal Parkinson's disease, such as an oculogyric crisis – extension of the head and rolling of the eyes – and a change in the sleep–wake cycle. This condition does respond to dopaminergic drugs.

Wilson's disease

Wilson's disease is an important disorder to distinguish from Parkinson's disease because the treatment is entirely different. Wilson's disease is an autosomal recessive disorder caused when a pair of weak genes is inherited, one from each parent. The illness results in an abnormality of copper metabolism and, in particular, the deposition of copper in certain tissues such as the liver, eyes and brain.

It may develop at any age from adolescence up to the age of 50 or so. For this reason patients who show parkinsonian symptoms under the age of 50 are usually investigated for the possibility of Wilson's disease. This is done relatively simply. Blood tests are checked for copper levels and ceruloplasmin (the protein that carries copper in the blood), the eyes are tested for copper deposition (sometimes this can be seen only with a special ophthalmologist's viewfinder) and the urine is checked for excess excretion of copper.

Treatment is usually successful in restoring normal health and involves giving tablets that increase the excretion of copper from the body and prevent damage to the tissues.

Neuroleptic tablets

Perhaps the most common cause of symptoms that mimic Parkinson's disease is a certain type of medication called a neuroleptic. Neuroleptic tablets, for example, haloperidol and chlorpromazine, are often given for major psychiatric disturbances such as schizophrenia, but they can also be used for patients with periods of confusion and abnormal behaviour. They can be given 'to calm a patient down'. So a doctor will ask a patient with parkinsonian symptoms about recent medication in case this is a cause.

The reason why neuroleptic tablets cause symptoms similar to Parkinson's disease is because in some patients they have the side effect of blocking dopamine receptors and so inducing a state similar to lack of dopamine. Fortunately the symptoms usually disappear when the tablets are stopped, although occasionally they persist. Another common feature of some neuroleptic tablets is that they cause orofacial dyskinesias – abnormal, often continuous, involuntary movements, particularly of the tongue and mouth. These often also disappear when the tablets are stopped, although sometimes it can take months or years – and occasionally they are permanent.

Needless to say, such neuroleptic tablets should not be taken by patients who have Parkinson's disease. Fortunately, there are now some new types of neuroleptic tablet that do not produce severe side effects and can be used in patients with Parkinson's disease. These include compounds such as olanzapine, clozapine and quetiapine.

Other medication

Certain other medications may sometimes produce a tremor. These include inhalers that are used for asthma – for example, salbutamol (Ventolin) – and some tablets used for epilepsy or migraine – for example, sodium valproate (Epilim).

Benign essential tremor

In patients who just have a tremor as their only symptom the diagnosis may be a condition called benign essential tremor. This runs in families in about half of those with the condition. It is the result of autosomal dominant inheritance (strong gene effect) and there is usually a history of a similar tremor in one or other parent or grandparent.

It differs from the tremor of Parkinson's disease in that it is often present from the beginning on both sides of the body and the patient does not have the tremor when at rest but only on going to do something. Furthermore, patients with benign essential tremor do not typically have features of stiffness or rigidity. Even so, it can sometimes be difficult to distinguish between Parkinson's disease and benign essential tremor.

Thyroid gland overactivity

Another cause of tremor that needs investigation is that caused by thyroid gland overactivity. This produces a fine tremor in which the amount of movement is small although it is present almost all the time. It is diagnosed by a simple blood test and can be treated in a relatively straightforward manner. Conversely, underactivity of the thyroid gland can result in slowness which can sometimes be confused with Parkinson's disease.

Conditions that can mimic Parkinson's disease

- Multiple system atrophy
- Progressive supranuclear palsy
- Postencephalitic parkinsonism
- Wilson's disease
- Neuroleptic tablets
- Other medication
- Benign essential tremor
- Thyroid gland overactivity

KEY POINTS

- The diagnosis is from clinical signs – if necessary, it can be supported by a scan

- A number of neurological conditions mimic Parkinson's disease – generally speaking, they do not respond well to dopamine drugs

- In some patients, blood tests, scans and other investigations are required to exclude other diagnoses

Drugs used in the treatment of Parkinson's disease

Mechanisms of drug action

As explained in an earlier chapter, nerve cells communicate using chemical messengers called neurotransmitters. These are passed from one nerve cell to another at connections between the two, called synapses. In Parkinson's disease there is loss of nerve cells that use dopamine as a neurotransmitter. There is also loss of other nerve cells that use different neurotransmitters, including acetylcholine and 5-hydroxytryptamine. This leads to a complex interaction between different neurotransmitters, resulting in increased sensitivity to some of them in Parkinson's disease patients.

There are many drugs that can help to alleviate the symptoms of Parkinson's disease and they work in several different ways. Dopaminergic drugs compensate for the loss of dopamine by increasing the brain's reserve of dopamine. Other drugs act as dopamine mimics and activate the receptors on the nerve cells that would have reacted with dopamine itself (dopamine agonists). Still others lower the heightened sensitivity of the Parkinson's disease brain to acetylcholine (anticholinergics). Finally, other medications can be used to block excitotoxicity (see page 37). Each of these mechanisms is discussed in turn below.

Drugs used in Parkinson's disease

Class of drug	Generic name	Proprietary name
Dopamine replacement (levodopa) combined with an enzyme inhibitor	Cobeneldopa Cocareldopa	Madopar Sinemet
Additional enzyme inhibitor	Entacapone	Comtess/Stalevo
Dopamine agonists	Apomorphine Bromocriptine Cabergoline Lisuride Pergolide Pramipexole Ropinirole	APO-go Parlodel Cabaser Lisuride Celance Mirapexin Requip
Monoamine oxidase inhibitors	Selegiline	Eldepryl, Zelapar
Anticholinergics	Benzhexol Orphenadrine	Broflex Biorphen, Disipal
Excitotoxicity blocker	Amantadine	Symmetrel

Levodopa
How does it work?

Levodopa was the first medication produced for Parkinson's disease after the discovery that dopamine levels were lower in the brain of patients with Parkinson's disease. Levodopa can be taken up by cells in the brain and converted into dopamine, which relieves the symptoms of Parkinson's disease. It can be taken by several different routes, although by mouth in a tablet or liquid form is the most common.

About 99 per cent of levodopa taken by mouth would be destroyed in the intestine by two enzymes – aromatic amino acid decarboxylase (AAAD) and catechol-O-methyl transferase (COMT). To reduce this, the levodopa tablets – that is, cobeneldopa and cocareldopa – include an inhibitor to block one of the enzymes that destroy levodopa. This increases the absorption of levodopa into the bloodstream, although the inhibitor is not completely effective and most of the levodopa is still destroyed in the intestine. An additional form of enzyme inhibitor, entacapone, is now available and this drug further decreases the destruction of levodopa in the gut. The use of the enzyme inhibitors also helps to reduce the side effects of levodopa such as nausea, vomiting and gastrointestinal upset.

Once in the bloodstream, the levodopa is carried to the brain where it is taken up by nerve cells that use dopamine as a neurotransmitter – the cells that are affected in Parkinson's disease. These remaining cells convert the levodopa to dopamine. The dopamine is then packaged into the nerve cells ready for use as a neurotransmitter, so overcoming the lack of dopamine caused by the death of many of the cells in the substantia nigra.

Levodopa can be taken up by nerve cells in the brain and converted into dopamine

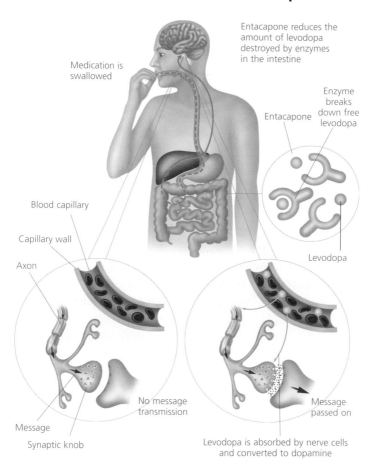

Entacapone reduces the amount of levodopa destroyed by enzymes in the intestine

Medication is swallowed

Enzyme breaks down free levodopa

Entacapone

Levodopa

Blood capillary

Capillary wall

Axon

No message transmission

Message passed on

Message

Synaptic knob

Levodopa is absorbed by nerve cells and converted to dopamine

Without levodopa

Nerve cell sends electrical signal along axon

There is insufficient neurotransmitter to cross the synapse

No message transmission

With levodopa

Message travels along axon to synaptic knob

Neurotransmitter crosses synapse

Receptor cells are activated

Message passed on

The 'wearing-off' effect

When a patient first starts levodopa, the effect is often dramatic with rapid and substantial improvement of parkinsonian symptoms such as stiffness and slow movements. In the early stages (the first couple of years) patients may need only two or three doses of levodopa a day. Later, however, each dose becomes a little less effective. This is probably not the result of any loss of effectiveness of levodopa, but rather the continued loss of nerve cells that are available to take up levodopa and convert it into dopamine. Thus, patients find that the benefit from each levodopa tablet does not last as long, and they begin to experience so-called 'wearing off' or 'off periods' in which symptoms such as weakness and immobility recur.

The 'wearing-off' effect can be avoided in several ways. The tablets come in different dosages, so the patient can simply take the same dose more often, maybe four to five times a day instead of two or three times. Another way is to change the tablet to one with a higher dose of levodopa. Alternatively, the patient can take a controlled-release form of levodopa, which helps eliminate peaks and troughs in the amount of the drug in the circulation.

Another approach introduced in the late 1990s is to add a COMT inhibitor to the levodopa tablets. This combination gets more levodopa to the brain – so it's a bit like increasing the dose of levodopa in the tablet. Tolcapone was the first COMT inhibitor used. After being withdrawn in 1998, it has now been reintroduced. Entacapone is currently used – it doesn't affect the liver, and seems to be an effective and safe form of treatment. Entacapone (like tolcapone) is effective only when combined with levodopa. A single tablet containing levodopa with entacapone, called Stalevo, has recently become available.

Side effects
Nausea
Virtually all medicines taken in tablet form have side effects and levodopa is no exception. Levodopa can sometimes cause nausea, vomiting or gastrointestinal upset, even though this is less now that an enzyme inhibitor for AAAD is always included. Some patients have nausea when they first start levodopa but it gradually wears off as the treatment is continued.

Sleepiness
Another side effect is sleepiness. Patients find that they fall asleep more easily during the day, sometimes at inappropriate times. This can be seen even in patients who are not on treatment for their Parkinson's disease, but is seen more commonly in those on levodopa or dopamine agonists. Some patients, particularly elderly ones, may have confusion or hallucinations when they take levodopa.

Dizziness
Levodopa can lower the blood pressure, particularly in response to a change in posture (postural hypotension) – for example, when you get out of bed or rise from a chair quickly, your body's natural response is to increase your blood pressure so enough blood still reaches your brain. Levodopa can sometimes interfere with this natural response and patients may feel a little light-headed or dizzy, or at worst faint, if they get up too quickly. This is usually most easily managed by changing posture more slowly, such as sitting on the side of the bed for a few

seconds before standing up or rising from a chair and waiting for a moment or two before walking away.

There are a few people who cannot tolerate levodopa and alternative treatments need to be tried.

Dyskinesias (involuntary movements)

One of the most significant limitations to the use of levodopa is the possibility of the side effect of dyskinesias (involuntary movements). These can be quite subtle in the beginning and may only be a slight twitch or writhing movement of the shoulder, arm or hand. As they become more noticeable with time so they become more troublesome and can occasionally be quite dramatic, causing grimacing and dramatic limb movements. These involuntary movements can affect any part of the body, including the mouth and tongue. People have great difficulty in suppressing them and find this side effect particularly troublesome in company. Unfortunately the dyskinesias are made worse by stress or anxiety.

Very often the dyskinesias occur at a time of day related to when levodopa tablets are taken, commonly about an hour and a half to two hours after taking a tablet – when there is most levodopa in the blood. The movements may last for 30 minutes or longer, and these are referred to as peak-dose dyskinesias. Sometimes the onset of dyskinesias is not so obviously associated with the timing of the levodopa dose – for example, some patients find that they develop relatively soon after taking a tablet. They then disappear but return as the effectiveness of the tablet wears off. These are called biphasic dyskinesias and are probably triggered by a particular concentration of levodopa in the blood.

The combination of dyskinesias and 'wearing off' is grouped under what is called the 'motor complications' of levodopa. These are estimated to occur in about half of all patients who have taken levodopa for as long as five years. Young-onset Parkinson's disease patients (those who develop the disorder before the age of 50) seem to be more likely to develop motor (movement) complications – about 70 per cent of such patients will have motor complications within three years of starting treatment with levodopa.

Quite why motor complications develop as a consequence of levodopa use is not known. As indicated above, the 'wearing off' is probably related to the underlying progression of the disease. It does not seem to be a toxic effect of the drug. Dyskinesias, it seems, are more related to the intermittent pattern of use of the drug and the consequent intermittent activation of the dopamine receptors in the brain. Also, the more advanced a patient's disease is when he or she starts levodopa, the more likely he or she is to develop dyskinesias.

In the light of these findings, various strategies have been developed to establish a long-term scheme for the management of Parkinson's disease patients. The aim is to prevent, or at least decrease, the risk of developing motor complications. The strategies are explained below.

Dopamine agonists
How do they work?
Dopamine agonists are drugs that have a similar effect to that of levodopa but a different mechanism of action: they lock on to dopamine receptors and therefore they substitute for dopamine. They are mostly prescribed as tablets but may also be taken by intravenous injection.

How dopamine agonists work

Dopamine agonists have a similar effect to levodopa but a different mode of action: they lock on to dopamine receptors and therefore substitute for dopamine.

Without dopamine agonist
Nerve cell sends electrical signal along axon

There is insufficient neurotransmitter to cross the synapse

No message transmission

With dopamine agonist
Message travels along axon to synaptic knob

Neurotransmitter crosses synapse

Receptor cells are activated

Message passed on

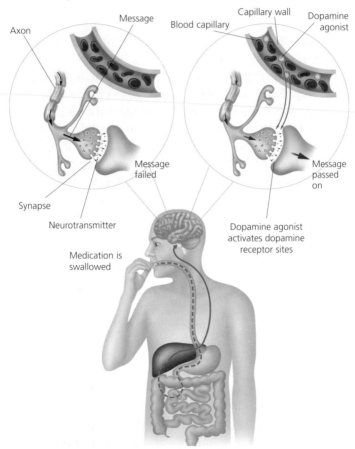

Dopamine agonists do not need to be converted by the brain but work directly by acting as a dopamine neurotransmitter. These drugs can control the symptoms of Parkinson's disease that result from lack of dopamine and so can be used to delay the need to prescribe levodopa. Dopamine agonists may be given together with levodopa, and therefore allow lower doses of levodopa to be used.

Dopamine agonists are particularly useful to control the stiffness and slowness of movement of Parkinson's disease. They may also be helpful in controlling the tremor of some patients.

A variety of dopamine agonists is available (see box on page 51). Those more recently developed act for longer and seem to be better tolerated. When a patient starts taking a dopamine agonist the initial dose will be very small, and the dose is then gradually increased over a period of a few weeks. This helps to prevent problems with nausea. If patients do develop nausea it usually wears off as the tablets are continued. Alternatively, an anti-nausea tablet, domperidone, can be given for the first two weeks when an agonist is introduced, and this prevents the nausea developing. It is important for the dopamine agonist dose to be gradually increased until an effective daily dose is reached.

The effectiveness of dopamine agonists can be comparable to levodopa if used at the right dose. An important advantage of dopamine agonists is that they appear to be significantly less likely to cause motor complications including 'wearing off' and dyskinesias. Several studies with dopamine agonists including cabergoline (Cabaser), ropinirole (Requip), pramipexole (Mirapexin) and pergolide (Celance) have all shown a significantly lower risk of dyskinesias developing in those patients initiated on the agonist compared with those started on levodopa. Indeed those patients who were able to take dopamine agonists alone for the relief of their Parkinson's disease symptoms had a very low rate of motor complications.

Two recent studies using either pramipexole (Mirapexin) or ropinirole (Requip) suggested that newly diagnosed patients who were started on one of these dopamine agonists had a slower rate of progression of their nerve cell loss than did those patients started on levodopa. This effect was assessed by using SPECT or PET scans to follow patients over two or four years from the start of their treatment. These results could support a neuroprotective effect for pramipexole and ropinirole. However, the results could also be explained by a potential toxic effect of levodopa or an effect of the drugs on the scans themselves, although there is little evidence currently to support these arguments. At present it is probably fair to say that the study results are exciting, but not conclusive of a neuroprotective effect.

Side effects

The range of side effects with dopamine agonists is similar to those for levodopa except that the risk for development of dyskinesias is lower. However, episodes of confusion or hallucinations are more common with dopamine agonists than levodopa. So dopamine agonists need to be used more cautiously in elderly people, who are more susceptible to these symptoms. Additional side effects with dopamine agonists may include some swelling of the ankles or blotchiness over the legs. These additional side effects rarely cause serious problems. Dopamine agonists may also be associated with sleepiness and some reports of sudden onset of sleep have been described. If you are affected by sleepiness, discuss it with your doctor and do not drive while affected. Pergolide has rarely been associated with fibrosis (stiffening) of heart valves.

Apomorphine

Apomorphine is a quick-acting, short-duration dopamine agonist that must be given by injection. It is extremely helpful for those patients who experience severe 'off' periods. The apomorphine dose is carefully regulated for each patient and can be given as an injection using a PenJet. This is relatively easy to perform and delivers a small dose of apomorphine subcutaneously (under the skin), from where it is rapidly absorbed. Benefits usually appear in about 10 minutes and can last from about 60 to 90 minutes. In some circumstances the apomorphine may best be given by subcutaneous injection using an infusion pump.

Anticholinergics

Anticholinergic tablets are designed to block the acetylcholine receptor on nerves that use this chemical as a neurotransmitter. Anticholinergics such as benzhexol and orphenadrine are still used in the management of Parkinson's disease and appear to be modestly effective. Their problem is that they are more frequently associated with side effects than dopamine agonists or levodopa. These side effects include dryness of the mouth and confusion, and they have to be used with caution in patients with glaucoma or men with prostatism. Anticholinergics do not, however, appear to be associated with a risk of dyskinesias.

Monomine oxidase inhibitors

Selegiline and rasagiline block the activity of an enzyme in the brain called monoamine oxidase B. As monoamine oxidase B destroys dopamine, by blocking its action dopamine lasts longer in the brain. Both drugs improve the symptoms of Parkinson's disease although their effect is relatively modest. They can be used alone or together with levodopa or dopamine agonists.

A few years ago there was a concern that patients treated with selegiline might have an increased mortality rate but careful studies since that time have shown that selegiline is not associated with any such risk and is a relatively safe and well-tolerated drug. In some patients however, selegiline can produce confusion.

Selegiline was one of the treatments used in a very large trial in the USA called DATATOP. This investigated whether selegiline or vitamin E might have some beneficial effect in slowing down the progression of Parkinson's disease. The results for selegiline were positive, although many have argued that the beneficial effects were not the result of any protection by selegiline on the nerve cells in the substantia nigra, but rather caused by a direct benefit in improving symptoms. Recent laboratory studies have suggested that some of the drugs that may be similar to selegiline may have some potential in slowing down Parkinson's disease.

Rasagiline is a new MAO-B inhibitor and is more potent than selegiline. It needs to be given only once a day. It has been shown to improve the symptoms of Parkinson's disease at all stages of the illness. The drug appears to be well tolerated with few side effects. Rasagiline is different from selegiline in that no part

How selegiline works

Selegiline blocks the activity of an enzyme in the brain that
destroys dopamine.

1. Message transmission

Message travels along axon to synaptic knob
Neurotransmitter crosses synapse
Receptor cells are activated
Message passed on

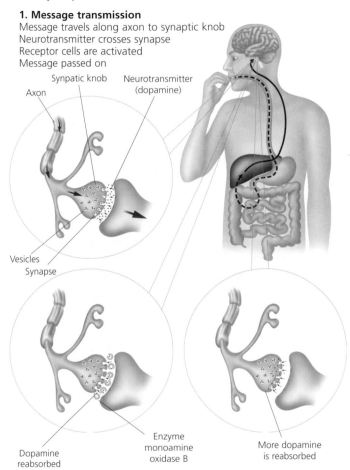

Synpatic knob

Neurotransmitter
(dopamine)

Axon

Vesicles

Synapse

Dopamine
reabsorbed

Enzyme
monoamine
oxidase B

More dopamine
is reabsorbed

2. After message transmission

Dopamine is either reabsorbed into
the synaptic knob or destroyed by
the enzyme monoamine oxidase B
in the synapse

3. With MAO-B inhibition

Selegiline and rasagiline blocks the
activity of the enzyme monoamine
oxidase B in the brain which
destroys dopamine so there is
more dopamine available

of the drug is metabolised to amphetamine. The amphetamine metabolites of selegiline may contribute to its side effect profile.

One study in Parkinson's disease patients has suggested that rasagiline may slow the progress of the illness. However, this study needs to be repeated before we can use rasagiline as 'europrotection' rather than just symptomatic treatment.

Amantadine

Amantadine is used to treat a variety of disorders including viral infections such as influenza. It gives some modest relief from the symptoms of Parkinson's disease. Again it is well tolerated but can induce some side effects, including a purplish rash on the legs. The beneficial effects of amantadine in Parkinson's disease patients do not seem to be permanent, and the effects of the tablets seem to wear off after about six to twelve months. Amantadine can reduce dyskinesias in some patients without making other symptoms worse.

There has been recent interest in whether amantadine and similar drugs may have some effect in slowing down Parkinson's disease. At present there are no data to support this.

Strategy for the treatment and management of Parkinson's disease
The importance of the individual

Although there is significant individual variability between patients diagnosed with Parkinson's disease, there are general principles that are useful to follow in developing a long-term strategy for the treatment of the disorder.

Inevitably, some patients may respond better to one drug than to another, even if of the same drug type, and it is sometimes necessary to change medications if a patient does not respond well or develops side effects. Inevitably, a patient's response to treatment can be evaluated only over several days or weeks, because drugs need time to act and there is often some day-to-day variation in response.

Immediate treatment

As mentioned previously, a diagnosis of Parkinson's disease does not necessarily result in immediate treatment. Traditionally, this has been dependent on the severity of the patient's symptoms and their effect on an individual's social life and employment. However, some argue that, although this may be a good strategy for levodopa – that is, delaying its introduction because of its potential risk of inducing motor (movement) complications – this same strategy does not necessarily apply to dopamine agonists. Indeed some neurologists now recommend that dopamine agonists can be introduced for the patient's benefit at the time of diagnosis. Nevertheless, considerable debate continues in this area and the decision on the timing of the start of treatment needs to be made following careful discussion between the patient and his or her doctor(s).

First-line therapy

Despite the above differences of opinion, many specialists feel that, once a patient develops symptoms sufficient to warrant therapy, it is best to introduce a dopamine agonist first unless there are good reasons to do otherwise. Dopamine agonists are effective and well tolerated in the great majority of patients and they have a distinct advantage over levodopa when given alone in their lack of long-term side effects, particularly in relation to dyskinesias and 'wearing off'. Nevertheless, there are some circumstances where it would seem more sensible to introduce levodopa – for example, in elderly people in whom the risk and relevance of long-term complications of levodopa may not necessarily be so important, and in those with some impairment of mental abilities.

Several studies have looked at the use of dopamine agonists as the first treatment of Parkinson's disease and these drugs appear to be capable of maintaining patients for several years, although not indefinitely. For instance, by about five years, up to 70 per cent of patients who were started on a dopamine agonist will have required some levodopa to be added to their medication. Nevertheless, 30 per cent of Parkinson's disease patients are still well maintained on an agonist alone.

Second-line therapy

If a patient is started on a dopamine agonist, the dose of this may need to be gradually increased over the years in order for the patient to continue to benefit from it. Nevertheless, at some point increasing the dose further will not lead to additional relief of symptoms or may even cause side effects. At this point most doctors would recommend adding in levodopa. If the dopamine agonist is continued it reduces the risk of complications with levodopa because a lower dose is needed.

Levodopa is generally introduced as a two or three times a day dose. As time goes by, both the frequency and the size of each dose may need to be increased. At some point during this process, a COMT inhibitor (entacapone) may be added to prolong the effect of levodopa. Some have suggested that the early use of a COMT inhibitor, indeed when levodopa is first introduced, may, by prolonging the action of levodopa, help to reduce the development of motor complications. This idea is now being tested in a trial and could be another important advance for patients.

The dyskinesias that develop in some patients taking levodopa can be troublesome. If they occur when levodopa is at its highest level in the blood it may be possible to find a dose and frequency of levodopa that produce less dyskinesia. Dopamine agonists can also produce dyskinesias, although whether they can do so when taken alone or require previous exposure to levodopa is not yet certain. So in someone with dyskinesias who is taking both types of drugs, a balance will have to be reached among doses of levodopa and agonist, the development of dyskinesias and the control of the symptoms of Parkinson's disease. As a general rule, at this stage of the disease, the more levodopa or agonist a patient takes, the more they are likely to experience dyskinesias. The less they take, the more likely they are to experience Parkinson's disease symptoms.

Another way to lessen dyskinesias is to add in cabergoline, a once-a-day, long-acting agonist. This drug can lessen dyskinesias by 'smoothing out' the stimulation of dopamine receptors over a 24-hour period. It can be taken with levodopa or given alone and allows the dose of levodopa to be reduced. It may also be used in conjunction with other dopamine agonists.

Taking medicines

Some patients find that their response to levodopa – and even to dopamine agonists – can depend very much on the timing of meals and doses. For example, a lot of protein in a meal can reduce the absorption of levodopa. So, some patients find that it is best to keep any heavy protein meal to the end of the day after the last dose. Dopamine agonists are probably best taken either 30 minutes before or 45 minutes after a meal. Thus manipulation of diet can sometimes produce some benefit in these fluctuations. You should speak to your state-registered dietitian about this.

Recently, amantadine (see page 64) has been shown to decrease the frequency and severity of dyskinesias at a fixed dose of levodopa in a proportion of patients with Parkinson's disease. This is worth trying if other techniques have failed.

Patients with extremely troublesome dyskinesias, as well as unpredictable freezing episodes or 'off' periods, may be helped by giving drugs by a tube directly into the stomach – for example Duodopa – via an injection or even by surgery.

Dopamine agonists, such as apomorphine, can be used in a pump system with a needle inserted just below the skin (subcutaneous infusion). This system needs to be set up and, at least at the beginning, supervised in hospital but patients or their carers may learn to change the needle and syringe pump. If used correctly, such an infusion can substantially improve parkinsonian symptoms as well as motor complications. For some patients this can be a long-term solution but for most it is only practicable over short periods.

Levodopa can now be given as a gel by a pump which connects to a tube that enters the stomach directly from the abdominal wall. This infusion can improve fluctuations but is suitable for only selected patients.

KEY POINTS

■ There are several types of drug which act in different ways to compensate for a lack of dopamine

■ The different types of drug can be used alone or in combination

■ Levodopa replaces lost dopamine; dopamine agonists mimic the action of dopamine

■ The strategy of management with drugs is tailored to the individual and changes as advances in medical science are made

Surgery for Parkinson's disease

The history of surgery

Some readers will be surprised to hear that surgery for patients with Parkinson's disease began as long ago as the first half of the twentieth century. Early procedures involved pallidotomy and thalamotomy. These involved destroying parts of the basal ganglia that were thought to exacerbate parkinsonian symptoms. At that time these operations carried a significant risk of side effects and so were abandoned when levodopa was first introduced.

Nowadays we recognise that there are limitations to levodopa therapy and there have been substantial advances in neurosurgery and ways in which the brain can be scanned. This has led to the modern development of surgery for patients with Parkinson's disease.

Pallidotomy

There are several types of procedure that may be undertaken. Pallidotomy is probably still the most frequent. This involves destroying part of the globus pallidus with an electric current or freezing, using a tiny probe carefully placed in the brain. Potential complications are related to the insertion of the probe into the brain, and can include haemorrhage or stroke, although this is rare, especially if the procedure is undertaken by an experienced neurosurgeon. Symptoms such as stiffness, rigidity, tremor and dyskinesias can be reduced on the opposite side of the body. If both sides are affected it is possible to have a pallidotomy on both sides, but the risk of complications is much greater, and may include problems with speech, swallowing and mental abilities.

Thalamotomy

A similar procedure, called a thalamotomy, may be undertaken on the thalamus and this is thought to be of particular help to patients with tremor.

Deep brain stimulation

More recently a new type of operation called 'deep brain stimulation' was pioneered by some neurosurgeons in France. It is now done in many centres around the world. A fine wire is inserted into the brain to a precise location and attached to a pacemaker. This produces a tiny electric current at the tip of the wire. The site at which the tip is inserted is obviously critical to the success. Two sites are currently chosen, either the subthalamic nucleus or the globus pallidus, and it is not yet clear which produces the best results. The wire is attached to a pacemaker, which is placed under the skin of the shoulder. Both the wire and pacemaker are left in; the pacemaker can be turned on or off by the patient.

Deep brain stimulation

A fine wire is inserted into a precise location in the brain and attached to a pacemaker to produce a tiny electrical stimulation at the tip of the wire.

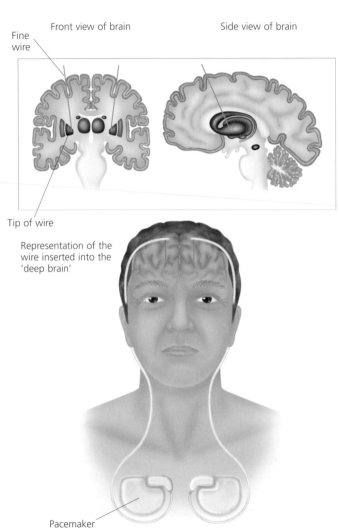

Front view of brain

Side view of brain

Fine wire

Tip of wire

Representation of the wire inserted into the 'deep brain'

Pacemaker

Symptoms of bradykinesia, rigidity and dyskinesia may be improved on the opposite side of the body. In contrast to pallidotomy, deep brain stimulation can be given to both sides of the brain without risk of significant side effects. It is associated with a very low risk of haemorrhage or stroke. Problems may arise with infection or breakage of the wire, but these are rare.

Deep brain stimulation must be undertaken by a team of doctors which includes an experienced neurosurgeon and those who can programme the pacemaker to stimulate the brain correctly.

Cell implants

Work is taking place to find a way to restore function to patients with Parkinson's disease by implanting cells into the damaged regions of the brain. Cells from a patient's adrenal medulla (which normally produces neuotransmitter substances including dopamine) have been tried but little improvement in symptoms was found.

Mixed results have been obtained with cells taken from the brain of aborted human fetuses. These cells develop into neurons of the type lost from the substantia nigra in Parkinson's disease. It is a very intricate procedure – great experience is required to obtain the cells at the correct stage of fetal development, keep them alive and inject them into exactly the right place in the brain. So far the results have been varied. Some groups have had spectacular successes in the control and even abolition of symptoms whereas others have had failures and complications with worsening of their symptoms. It is clear that this technique is still being refined and should be undertaken only by groups with considerable experience and some success.

It has been possible to examine a few brains of patients who have died for another reason a year or two after they received fetal implants. It was found that the fetal cells had not only survived but had also connected with the patient's own brain cells and provided a source of dopamine. These results are extremely encouraging. Nevertheless, it seems likely that fetal brain implants will remain rare specialist procedures, not least because of practical and ethical problems in obtaining the fetal material.

Work is now taking place to develop human cells that can be grown in a laboratory and will produce dopamine, perhaps by altering the cell's DNA. These cells may then be put into a special type of capsule that protects them but allows the dopamine to leave. These capsules may be microscopic and suitable for inserting into the same area of the brain as fetal implants.

Stem cells from embryos

A further area of research is the use of stem cells from human embryos. These cells are at an immature, early stage of development and, with the correct genetic signal, can change into any type of cell, including nerve cells. This is what happens normally after fertilisation – the few cells that grow from the fertilised egg go on to develop into all the different types of cell that form a baby. Each cell in your body has the genetic information to become any type of cell – it just depends which genes are active or 'switched on'. It is hoped that we can find out how to switch on the genes that convert stem cells into neurons for implantation to improve Parkinson's disease. This research is only at the earliest stages, so it will be several years before this therapy can be successfully applied. All cell implant procedures are still only at the experimental stage and are not available as treatments.

Growth factors

Growth factors are molecules that can be obtained from a variety of different cell types in the body. They occur naturally and are designed to encourage the growth and maturation of cells. Brain-derived and glial cell (a type of cell in the brain) derived growth factors have both been used with success in models (animals such as rats with Parkinson's disease-like symptoms) of Parkinson's disease and in some Parkinson's disease patients. The method of delivery may involve direct infusion into the brain, or possibly implantation of cells able to manufacture these growth factors. This research is exciting but at an early stage. If further trials support the use of growth factors, they may become a useful addition to Parkinson's disease treatment.

KEY POINTS

- Modern surgical techniques can provide benefits for some people and risks are reducing all the time

- Deep brain stimulation is a skilled technique that is becoming more widely available

- Research on cell implants is very active and may provide relief in future

Frequently asked questions about Parkinson's disease

Why me?

Patients often wonder why they have developed Parkinson's disease and whether something that they have done during their life, for example, their job or diet, may have contributed. In general, it is extremely rare for anything that a person does to predispose them to develop Parkinson's disease. Certainly, there is nothing in the diet that we know of that can increase an individual's risk. Other environmental factors identified so far also seem to have a very weak link to the cause.

It may be that, with time, we will discover more about what predisposes patients to Parkinson's disease. Even in those with a family history, unless the family history is very strong with multiple individuals in each generation being affected, then the chances of a genetic contribution are small. Certainly, those patients who have one or more brothers or sisters with

Parkinson's disease, but whose parents were normal, might have inherited the so-called weak gene effect from each parent which, when together, can produce the illness. An example of this is the parkin gene (see page 26).

Overall, the answer to this question is most often 'We don't know'.

What is the cause?

As suggested above, although the last 10 years have seen significant advances in our understanding of some of the causes of Parkinson's disease and also how the brain may be damaged during the course of the illness, we are still far from knowing all the different causes and their details.

Is it inherited – will I pass it on?

There is a genetic predisposition for Parkinson's disease in a minority of patients. Those who have a parent, brother or sister with Parkinson's disease are at a slightly increased risk of developing the disorder but this risk is small, so the answer to the question 'will I pass it on?' must be 'highly unlikely'. The only exception to this is those rare families where multiple generations and several members of each generation are affected.

How long ago did this start?

Patients are often aware of symptoms of Parkinson's disease creeping up on them and, looking back, can see that it may have been 12 to 18 months after the symptoms began before they sought medical advice. A patient's partner may also be a good guide in assessing how long the symptoms have been present. They are often good at picking up changes in the behaviour pattern or mobility of their partner even before the patient.

But the damage to brain cells starts before symptoms appear. For most Parkinson's disease patients, damage to the nerve cells probably began some five to ten years before the diagnosis was made. Inevitably, this is a generalisation and there are exceptions. For instance, those individuals who inherit a strong mutant gene from one parent (for example, alpha-synuclein) or those with two mutant weak genes (for example, parkin) have had the genetic defect since birth, and the damage to brain cells may have started several decades before the diagnosis in their 40s or 50s. Other individuals, who were exposed to the MPTP poison, developed Parkinson's disease within seven to fourteen days.

What should I expect?

The course of Parkinson's disease is very variable and it really is true to say that each patient is different. There are important biological reasons for this difference. For instance, the genetic make-up of an individual, personality and general health all affect the way the symptoms of Parkinson's disease might develop. Good general health and a positive attitude seem to have a significantly beneficial effect on the future of a Parkinson's disease patient.

The damage to nerve cells is ongoing but the progression rate varies considerably between patients. Many patients appear to go a number of years without any significant change in their Parkinson's disease. A few patients appear to progress more rapidly. At present it is not possible to slow down or stop the process of Parkinson's disease but there is a huge amount of research into this, some with significant success.

Thus, in answer to the question, it is important to emphasise the variability of the illness, and for the patient to understand the importance of a positive mental attitude and a healthy lifestyle. A further cause for optimism is the significant medical advances being made currently to slow down the illness.

Do I need to start treatment now?

Medication will help to relieve your symptoms, particularly those that are related to your lack of dopamine. So you will probably want to start when your symptoms interfere with your life – either socially or at work.

If you are a young-onset patient with a high-pressure job, you may need to begin treatment early so you can stay at work and function relatively normally. If you have retired and are not particularly troubled by your symptoms of tremor or stiffness, you may be able to delay starting treatment.

You should discuss in detail with your doctor when best to start treatment. It is understandable that you may want to delay medication but, if your lifestyle is significantly impaired, your doctor may ask you to reconsider this carefully. Some doctors prefer to delay levodopa treatment because of the potential side effects in the long term. Other doctors think that the motor complications of levodopa do not develop significantly sooner as a result of early introduction of this therapy.

When considering whether to start treatment, it is important to realise that not all the symptoms of Parkinson's disease will improve with levodopa or dopamine agonists. Constipation and some postural changes, for instance, may not necessarily improve so again this aspect needs to be discussed with your doctor, who will be able to suggest suitable treatments for these conditions.

What treatment should I start on?

Once you agree to medical treatment, there are various options. To some extent the choice depends on your particular characteristics.

Many specialists now agree that, unless there is a good reason to do otherwise, it is best to start with a dopamine agonist. They are easy to use, do not usually have troublesome side effects and give good relief of symptoms without the long-term motor (movement) complications associated with levodopa.

There are several dopamine agonists to choose from. The more recently introduced ones are the most widely used, including pramipexole, ropinirole, cabergoline and pergolide. As indicated in the chapter on treatment (see page 50), these tablets are usually started at a small dose and gradually increased. Your symptoms and adjustments to your lifestyle can be maintained at a steady state on dopamine agonists, often for a number of years, but may eventually require additional therapy in the form of levodopa.

However, if your risk of long-term motor complications seems less of a problem, for instance, if you are elderly or have a significant medical condition, it may be better for you to start on levodopa.

Your doctor may choose to start you on anticholinergics or selegiline. They are still often used as the first therapy after diagnosis. Selegiline gives some symptom relief and can delay the requirement for additional dopaminergic therapy.

Remember that advances are constantly being made in the treatment of Parkinson's disease and the advice given above may need to be modified with the introduction of new drugs.

If I take treatment, what symptoms will improve?

You will receive benefit only if you are taking an adequate amount of either a dopamine agonist or levodopa. Your doctor will adjust the dose carefully and it may take a few weeks to get it right.

The medication is most likely to improve symptoms that are caused by lack of dopamine in the brain. Most relief is found for stiffness and slowness (rigidity and bradykinesia). Tremor improves in some patients but not all. Symptoms such as constipation, postural instability, sweating disturbances, excess salivation and falls are not much affected.

If I don't take medication, what will happen?

This depends on what stage you are at. If you have not yet started treatment you will not have derived any benefit from the drugs used in Parkinson's disease. This may be because you and your doctor have decided that the time is not yet right to begin treatment.

If you have started treatment and benefited, then stopping the tablets will mean that your symptoms will usually reappear within a few days and may well be worse than before you started treatment. If levodopa or dopamine agonists are to be stopped, it is important that this is done gradually and not suddenly.

What can I do to help myself?

A positive attitude to Parkinson's disease and its treatment is important and helps you and your close ones to cope.

Exercise is important because it will help keep the joints and muscles supple and maintain strength. Naturally, the ability of a patient to exercise will vary from one to another. Some are able to go on a formal exercise programme whereas others organise a regular half-hour walk once or twice a day. Some patients find that an exercise bicycle helps and is convenient.

Physiotherapy is also important and most patients can benefit from being taught a programme of exercises. This initially needs to be given under the supervision of a qualified physiotherapist, but, once you have learnt the exercises, you can do them regularly at home.

You may be concerned about your illness and being in public but try to avoid social isolation – it can be very bad for you and your family. You should try as much as possible to maintain your normal level of social activity. Most people you meet will be very helpful, sympathetic and encouraging about Parkinson's disease. You may need a bit of cajoling in order to go out, but being among friends in public will often help you feel much more relaxed and happy.

There are no specific dietary changes that have been proved to help your symptoms. However, if you are taking levodopa, especially if you have been taking it for several years, you may have to be careful about when you eat protein. This is because a lot of protein in your meal can reduce your absorption of levodopa. If this happens, you can adjust the protein in your meals – perhaps by eating a light breakfast and lunch and having your main meal in the evening.

Most people benefit from finding out more about the disease and its treatment. The management of Parkinson's disease should be a partnership of your family, yourself and your doctor. You have priority in all decisions but it is often helpful to discuss important matters together – and to do this you need a good general knowledge of Parkinson's disease. Hopefully this book will go some way to providing that.

Will it shorten my life?

Before the introduction of levodopa, Parkinson's disease was associated with a reduction in life expectancy. However, since the widespread use of levodopa and other modern therapies, such as the dopamine agonists, Parkinson's diseases does not appear to affect a patient's life span significantly. You should look forward to a relatively normal life span with a good quality of life.

Does it affect my thinking and memory?

If you have Parkinson's disease, you may sometimes have problems with confusion or hallucinations. These may come from your medication or may be related to your brain cell dysfunction. They are usually only a problem in advanced cases. Unfortunately, levodopa or dopamine agonists do not improve this type of problem and can sometimes make it worse. Significant problems with thinking and memory, or with dementia, should call into question the diagnosis of pure Parkinson's disease, particularly if they occur at an early stage. Many of the disorders that look like Parkinson's disease are associated with significant problems with thinking and memory.

Many patients with Parkinson's disease become depressed. This is a natural reaction to an illness and has, in some studies, been estimated to occur in up to 75 per cent of patients with the illness. Often this goes undiagnosed and patients sometimes feel that it is just part of the illness. This is not so, however, and the depression deserves treatment in its own right. Importantly, significant depression can result in poor memory and problems with thinking and so effective treatment of depression can result not only in improvement of the patient's mood, but also in their thinking. The treatment for depression in Parkinson's disease is the same as the treatment that is routinely given for this problem – usually a choice between some form of psychotherapy and antidepressant drugs.

Can I continue to work?

There is no reason why you shouldn't continue to work. Many patients from a whole variety of occupations are able to continue their work almost as normal. Some of them require medication in order to help them stay at work, and there are many benefits of staying at work. It boosts your morale, keeps social contact and also maintains the morale of your family, as well of course as contributing to the finances.

If you're retired and have a part-time job, there's no reason why Parkinson's disease should interfere with this. However, the nature of your work may mean that it is difficult for you to continue if your symptoms are significant or if your work is in a hazardous environment. Those who work in stressful professions find that their symptoms can worsen. But, even for such people, effective treatment can help them to continue to work for several years.

Can I drive?

Many, if not most, patients with Parkinson's disease continue driving.

Once you have been diagnosed, you have to write to the DVLA (address in your driving licence) for their records. They will send you a simple questionnaire and your general practitioner may also be sent a simple form. For most patients this is all that is required and they can continue driving, although they may need to renew their licence more regularly simply in order to keep the DVLA informed. You must also notify your insurance company.

If you or your partner becomes concerned about your ability to drive, you can contact the DVLA and have a driving assessment. There are several such assessment centres in the UK, although there is a waiting list, so it may take a few weeks or months to organise.

As mentioned above (see page 60), levodopa or dopamine agonists may cause sedation. Sometimes this can result in you falling asleep in inappropriate circumstances. If you do feel sleepy, you must not drive and should wait until you've had a nap and feel perfectly alert. If you are worried about this, you should talk to your general practitioner or specialist. The rules regarding driving while taking certain types of medication for Parkinson's disease vary around the world.

Where can I get more information?

There are several important sources of information. You may find some better than others, depending on your circumstances.

One is your GP. He or she is often the first to suspect or diagnose Parkinson's disease and can be a very useful source of information. Also, together with your consultant, your GP will help you manage your disease over the years.

Your consultant is another important source of information. Consultants who look after Parkinson's disease may be neurologists or elderly care physicians (geriatricians). Those who have a particular interest in Parkinson's disease (movement disorder specialists) often run specialist clinics for patients.

The best way to get information from a GP or specialist is to write things down and take the list with you. Too often, when asked if they would like to ask any questions, patients find that their queries evaporate! Having a brief list of points and questions to be covered helps you and your doctor.

There are an increasing number of Parkinson's disease nurse specialists throughout the country. If you have one in your area, they can be an important source of information and support. For more on their role, see page 91.

You can find an enormous amount of information on the internet – and in newspapers and magazines. Many patients come to my clinic with cuttings and ask what I think about a particular tablet or treatment. This is a good thing – it allows patients with Parkinson's disease to have a balanced view of certain types of treatment that may be sensationalised in the popular press.

The Parkinson's Disease Society (PDS) plays a critical and important role for anyone with this disorder. The PDS is the only UK charity that exists to help all people living with Parkinson's disease. It provides education, care, information and research. The Society has a UK-wide network of branches, which provide advice, support and activities. You can get details of your local branch by calling the PDS National Office. There is a national network for young-onset patients with some local branches too. The PDS National Office address and contacts are given at the end of this book. It is an important source of information, advice and support, and I encourage all patients to join.

Will there be a cure?

I am sure that modern medicine will find a cure for Parkinson's disease and I am optimistic that this will be developed over the next 20 years. Historically, Parkinson's disease treatment has been considered to work only for the symptoms of the disorder and not to affect the underlying cause or the progression of the disease. Obviously improving the symptoms of a patient and restoring function and quality of life are very important. Nevertheless, the development of drugs that may slow down the course of the illness will be critically important. It may be that some of the drugs currently in use to improve the symptoms may actually slow down the progression of the disease as well.

The new types of treatment currently under development will probably lead to a cure. These include the so-called neuroprotective drugs, or neuro-rescue treatments, aimed at improving the functioning of sick or damaged neurons in the substantia nigra, and also preventing additional damage to those that are still intact. Such treatments currently being tested are medical – that is, will be given in tablet form – and this obviously will allow them to be accessible to all patients.

The other important route to a cure is by finding out more about the cause of Parkinson's disease.

Substantial advances have been made over the last 10 years and the rate of advancement is increasing all the time. It is for this reason that I am confident that a cure will be found.

However, a note of caution is required. A cure will be found only with sufficient research and resources being dedicated to Parkinson's disease. As a Parkinson's disease patient, you and your family can participate in this effort and often the best way to do so is through the Parkinson's Disease Society.

Can 'alternative' medicine help?

Traditional treatment for Parkinson's disease is based on a scientific understanding of what is chemically wrong with the brain that produces the symptoms of the disorder. Medication is to restore the missing chemicals as much as possible, and additional types of treatment such as physiotherapy and occupational therapy are to maintain function.

When patients ask about 'alternative' treatment they usually mean homoeopathic treatments, herbal remedies or acupuncture. At a personal level, I have no difficulty with a patient using such treatments. However, as a doctor I would prefer to see such treatments prove themselves in a tried and tested manner. I am always concerned when patients are asked to pay a significant amount of money for 'alternative' treatments that have not been scientifically proven to work.

It is often best to discuss with your doctor what alternative treatments you may wish to use, particularly as some of the herbal remedies may contain compounds that could interfere with tablets used for Parkinson's disease.

Are there any drug trials that I can take part in?

New treatments for Parkinson's disease are constantly being tested. Before they can be licensed it must be proved that they relieve the symptoms of Parkinson's disease in a better way than existing therapy.

All new drugs undergo a thorough period of testing in trials. These are usually undertaken by specialists in the field of Parkinson's disease. If you want to take part in a trial, discuss it with the specialist running the trial. He or she will probably talk to you about the trial and give you some leaflets. This will tell you what is being looked for, what the potential benefits might be and what possible side effects there may be to any new type of treatment.

Such trials are critically important because they are necessary before a new form of treatment can be used routinely. It is testimony to the helpfulness of patients with Parkinson's disease and their families that so many new drugs have been introduced – they cannot be developed without the help of patients. For advice on participating in trials contact the PDS (see 'Useful information' on page 113).

Living with Parkinson's disease

The importance of support

The quality of life of someone with Parkinson's disease depends on many factors. There is an increasing amount of support available aimed at helping to maintain or improve that quality. Parkinson's disease nurse specialists have proved valuable as a source of advice, support and education, and as a link to other services such as rehabilitation therapies.

The role of the Parkinson's disease nurse specialist

Parkinson's disease nurse specialists are based either in the community or in a hospital. They have been increasing in number since 1992, when the role was initiated through the Parkinson's Disease Society with the help of several pharmaceutical companies. There are now about 190 nationwide, although there is not as yet one in every area.

They are registered nurses with broad experience in neurology or care of elderly people and with

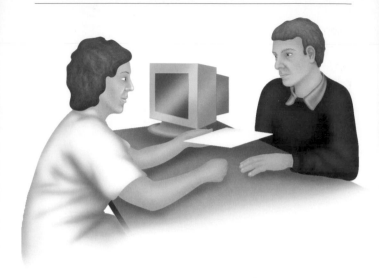

Parkinson's disease nurse specialists are a valuable source of advice, support and education, and as a link to other useful therapies.

specialised training in the management of Parkinson's disease. Their work involves assessing individual care needs, promoting each person's quality of life, and preventing or minimising the complications associated with Parkinson's disease.

Some of these complications can include fluctuations in mobility, urinary problems, constipation, depression, sexual dysfunction and side effects of medication. The Parkinson's disease nurse specialist can help by giving direct advice and perhaps referring to other professionals for more specific help.

When a patient receives the diagnosis of Parkinson's disease, it can be very bewildering and stressful – not only for that individual, but also for his or her friends and family. There is usually a period of uncertainty and fear of what the future may hold, and many questions arise. The Parkinson's disease nurse specialist can spend time with the patient at this crucial stage, listening to his or her concerns, providing reliable, up-to-date information, education and counselling. They can help to establish an appropriate plan of care, with ongoing contact. Just knowing that there is a professional with an in-depth knowledge of Parkinson's disease, at the end of a phone, can be very reassuring for the patient and the family.

Throughout the different stages of the disease, the Parkinson's disease nurse specialist can help to alleviate a patient's stress and anxiety in the management of the complications in Parkinson's disease. Other information on voluntary services, support services and organisations can also be supplied.

Together, your doctor and the Parkinson's disease nurse specialist provide a holistic ('whole body') approach to the health of each patient through physical, social and psychological support. They can act as the patient's advocate and provide a comprehensive and patient-centred service. The aim is to help each person with Parkinson's disease maintain his or her independence and ultimately to be in control of their condition.

Rehabilitation therapies for Parkinson's disease

Having Parkinson's disease can interfere with many day-to-day activities. The aim of therapies is to ease these difficulties by helping you to learn the knowledge and skills that you need to continue all your previous activities, whether at work or in the home, during leisure, social and family time. The three main therapies that are readily available are:

- physiotherapy
- occupational therapy
- speech and language therapy.

Physiotherapy
What are physiotherapists?

Physiotherapists will look at the difficulties that you may have with your movement and general mobility. They aim to help you achieve the greatest level of activity using the best quality of movement possible. They will teach you how to manage the physical aspects of your Parkinson's disease.

Qualified physiotherapists will be members of the Chartered Society of Physiotherapy. Like doctors, physiotherapists specialise in different areas of physiotherapy and not all physiotherapists have

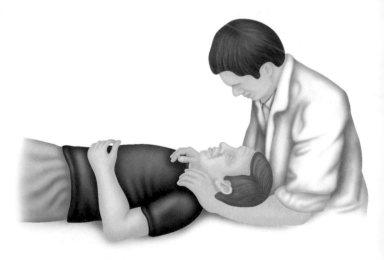

Physiotherapists will try to help you with difficulties that you may have with your movement and general mobility.

expertise in neurological disorders or Parkinson's disease. Physiotherapists interested in neurological disorders will be senior (not junior or basic grade) and are often called neurophysiotherapists. They may be members of the ACPIN (Association of Chartered Physiotherapists with an Interest in Neurology) or have done further specialist training.

What sorts of problems can physiotherapy help?

Physiotherapy is about learning how to move more normally and with less effort. It is not about routine exercise or regular treatment to prevent deterioration, but about learning skills and techniques to make coping with your Parkinson's disease easier.

Parkinson's disease can make automatic tasks, such as tying a tie or doing up shoe laces, slower. Certain techniques can improve this including learning strategies such as talking through a task while doing it or relying on visual targets to improve performance. These approaches are known as cueing. Sometimes splitting the movement up into a number of steps, or doing the task in a new way, can help. Physiotherapists can help teach all these techniques.

Parkinson's disease is also associated with stiffness and poor posture. Initially this is the result of the way Parkinson's disease affects movement, but later on the posture becomes habitual and muscles and joints become stiffer. Physiotherapists can work to relieve this muscle and joint stiffness.

As movements become more difficult, it is easy to become unfit. Physiotherapists can advise you about appropriate exercise – for example, Alexander technique or swimming.

Occuptional therapy
What are occupational therapists?

Having Parkinson's disease may mean that you may have problems with practicalities of daily life, such as looking after yourself and your family, or with work or leisure. It may also be difficult to get to the places you need to, both around the home and in the community. Occupational therapists (OTs) will work with you to identify your particular areas of difficulty and devise an individual treatment programme to help you overcome these problems.

Qualified occupational therapists will be state registered and may have either a diploma (DipCOT) or

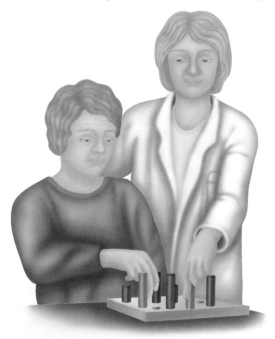

Occupational therapists can help identify, and suggest solutions to, problems that you may be having with everyday life.

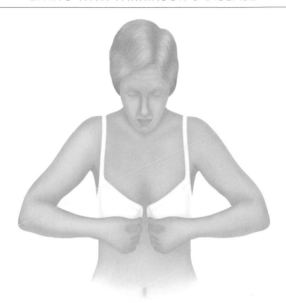

Getting dressed is easier with a bra that fastens at the front.

a degree (BSc(Hons) OT). Like physiotherapists, occupational therapists specialise in different areas. Occupational therapists interested in neurological disorders may be members of NANOT (National Association of Neurological OTs), or have done further specialist training.

What sorts of problems can occupational therapy help?

Occupational therapists help people with Parkinson's disease and their families to identify problems, which are impacting on their lifestyle, and to minimise the effect that these problems are having.

Like physiotherapists, occupational therapists may teach you to use new strategies when performing familiar tasks, such as getting dressed.

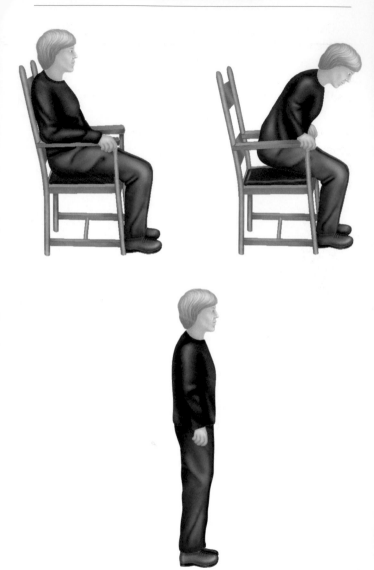

Occupational therapists may teach you new strategies to overcome
familiar tasks – for instance getting up from a chair.

Occupational therapists may provide or suggest simple equipment that makes performing a particular task easier, for example, using an electric can opener or a kettle tipper, or providing a chair raise. They may also provide advice about adaptations to your home, and how to fund these. Examples of simple adaptations include removing loose rugs and floor covers that may cause you to trip, or providing grab rails. Bigger adaptations include level access shower facilities, or stair lifts.

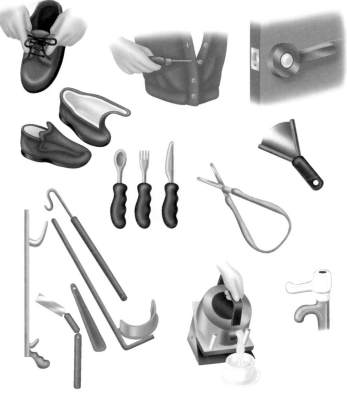

Household gadgets can help you around the home.

Many people with Parkinson's disease find day-to-day routines more effortful, and may experience fatigue. Occupational therapists will work with you to find daily and weekly routines that minimise effort and allow you to continue the activities that are most important to you.

Occupational therapists can also provide you with advice about resources that allow you to continue to work, to use transport, leisure and other community services, so that your life within the community remains as active as possible.

Speech and language therapy
What are speech and language therapists?
Speech and language therapists are involved in the assessment and treatment of people with communication and/or swallowing disorders. Qualified speech and language therapists are members of the Royal College of Speech and Language Therapy and will have a BSc(Hons) degree.

What sorts of problems can speech and language therapy help?
About half of people with Parkinson's disease develop some communication difficulties. These include slurred speech, quiet speech, poor expression, and speaking either too quickly or very slowly. Other communication difficulties might include difficulty with writing, limited facial expression and body language.

A speech and language therapist will work with a person with Parkinson's disease and, where appropriate, with the family or carers. They identify where the difficulties impact on lifestyle, for example, when using the telephone, or when speaking in public at meetings

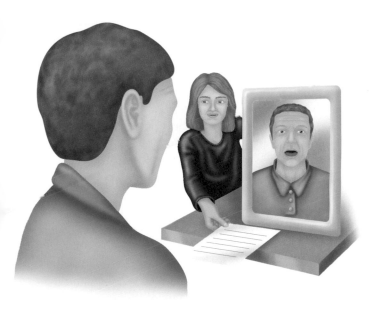

Speech and language therapists assess and treat people with communication and/or swallowing difficulties.

or in shops. Therapy can include exercises that work on improving voice loudness and therefore intelligibility of speech. Some people may find using a voice amplifier helpful.

The types of swallowing problems encountered by people with Parkinson's disease include difficulty controlling saliva, difficulty chewing harder foods and slowness to swallow. Some people may experience coughing or choking episodes while eating. The speech and language therapist will assess the swallow and provide advice on the easiest food and drink consistencies and the safest approach to eating and drinking.

When should I see any of these therapists?

Most physiotherapists believe that they should see people with Parkinson's disease early after diagnosis so that they understand the role of physiotherapy, what it can and can't do, and to prevent any unnecessary complications, such as poor posture, developing. Thereafter patients should be able to access physiotherapy when they identify a change in mobility which is limiting day-to-day activity.

You should ask to see an occupational therapist if you feel that your Parkinson's disease is impacting on any area of your everyday life.

You should ask to see a speech and language therapist if you feel that your Parkinson's disease is affecting your speech or swallowing even in a very minor way. It is often easier to learn compensatory techniques when the speech and swallowing problems are relatively mild, so early contact is advisable.

How do I get referred to a therapist?

Your family doctor or consultant usually makes the referral to therapists. In some areas the Parkinson's disease nurse specialist may also be able to make a referral.

Therapists work in a number of different settings. They may be based in a community health-care setting, in an acute hospital (outpatients or day hospital) or in Social Services. Each of these settings will have a slightly different perspective and approach, although all will have some overlap with each other.

Generally speaking, if you are seen in the outpatient department of an acute district hospital, most of your treatment will focus on learning new skills and techniques that you can practise in the hospital department and then try out at home. Community rehabilitation teams will tend to see you in your own home and look at task performance in your own environment. Social Services often provide equipment and suggest adaptations.

Being referred to a therapist in the wrong setting can be a frustrating experience. If you want to learn a technique for getting in and out of the bath but don't want bathing aids cluttering up your bathroom, you need referral to a community-based occupational therapist or physiotherapist – not one based in outpatients at your local hospital, or in a busy Social Services department who will provide a bath-board! For this reason, it is important to be clear about the type of intervention that you want.

What can I expect from my therapist?

You can expect your therapist to spend time with you identifying the areas that you are finding difficult and would like to change. You can then expect a period of treatment or intervention aimed at improving the difficulties that you have identified. A typical treatment course would be once a week for six weeks, but may be shorter. At the end of this time you would be discharged, ideally with some clear guidelines about when you should be reassessed.

What will my therapist expect from me?

It is easier for therapists to work with people who have clear ideas of what they want to change and why. It is therefore worth thinking about this before you meet your therapist. Many therapists will ask you to perform some type of exercise programme at home to build on what you have learnt in therapy sessions and, as far as possible, to transfer what you have learnt in therapy sessions to everyday life.

Over time you may see a number of different therapists in a number of settings. It is very helpful if you can keep a list of names, departments and contact numbers for all the therapists whom you have met. This helps therapists from different teams and specialities talk to each other and prevent work being duplicated.

Rehabilitation or multidisciplinary therapy

The therapies discussed here are often complementary to each other, as well as to medical and surgical interventions, because they individually work on different components of health and disease, or on similar components in a different way. You will often find the best results are obtained when therapists work together with you to find the best solution to a problem.

For example, although both physiotherapists and occupational therapists may work to improve bed-to-chair transfers, they will approach this goal in different manners and with different overall aims. The physiotherapist aims to increase muscular strength and flexibility with specific exercises, as well as teaching better movement strategies. Their overall aim is to enable the patient to get out of the chair as independently as possible. The occupational therapist, on the other hand, may assess the height and stability of the chair that the person is transferring from, teach movement, cueing and concentration strategies, and also look at the activities the person is going to undertake when he or she has got out of the chair.

Many therapists work in multi-disciplinary teams and

use a number of different approaches to managing a single problem. These therapists may form a community rehabilitation team or be based in a Parkinson's disease day hospital. If the therapists do not work in a team, a key worker may be needed to balance and coordinate care and this person is most commonly the Parkinson's disease nurse specialist.

KEY POINTS

- Parkinson's disease nurse specialists can provide support and advice and be a key link to other services

- Physiotherapists teach you how to manage your movement difficulties

- Occupational therapists give you practical solutions to everyday problems

- Speech and language therapists help with communication and swallowing

Future prospects

Huge investment in terms of money and effort is made into curing Parkinson's disease. The advances in our understanding of the causes of Parkinson's disease and ways in which we can treat patients have progressed rapidly over the last 10 years. This pace of change will only increase and will create numerous opportunities for improving the life of patients with Parkinson's disease.

Medical treatment
Symptom relief

Several new drugs are under development to improve the symptoms of Parkinson's disease. Drugs shortly to be released include a new monoamine oxidase B inhibitor (rasagiline). In clinical trials, this drug has proved to be effective in improving symptoms of early and more advanced Parkinson's disease. It appears to be safe and well tolerated. New dopamine agonists may shortly become available, in particular new formulations of dopamine agonists, including once-a-day preparations and skin-patch formulations. New studies will also look at how best to use some of our current treatments. For instance, there may be an opportunity for Stalevo (levodopa/carbidopa/entacapone) use to reduce the risk of motor complications developing when compared with levodopa. An important area for drug development is in the treatment of the non-motor (movement) symptoms of Parkinson's disease. This will be an area of intense activity over the next few years, and will probably see the introduction of entirely novel therapy for Parkinson's disease.

Neuroprotection

Slowing down or preventing the progression of Parkinson's disease, as well as reversing its symptoms, remains the ultimate goal for drug development in Parkinson's disease. Drugs such as dopamine agonists, rasagiline and coenzyme Q10 have all shown benefit in patients, with some suggestion that they might slow down the progression of the disease. However, these trials are at a preliminary stage, and cannot be interpreted as clearly showing disease modification. Future studies with these and other drugs have already started and the results are awaited with interest.

Surgery

At present, surgery remains a late option for patients with Parkinson's disease. However, preliminary trials with the infusion of growth factors such as glial cell-derived nerve factor (GDNF) or brain-derived nerve factor (BDNF) have shown some promise. These trials need to be extended to confirm benefit. Trials using fetal transplants have so far not shown clear advantages. However, research in this area is continuing, and future studies may be more promising. Another area of importance to the treatment of Parkinson's disease is the development of stem cell research. These are cells in the body that can be treated in such a way as to develop into neurons, including dopaminergic neurons. Theoretically, if implanted into the brain, these cells might take over the function of the neurons lost in Parkinson's disease. This research is again at a very early stage, but advances are already being made at a rapid rate.

Finally, cell capsules – that is, cells capable of releasing dopamine and enclosed in a protective capsule – could be inserted into the brain to substitute for the release of dopamine by the patient's brain.

As can be seen from the above there is an immense amount of promising research which should offer Parkinson's disease patients great optimism for the future.

Glossary

Agonists: agents that drive or stimulate the working of the site or receptor on which they act. By contrast, antagonists block or inhibit function.

Akinesia: loss of deliberate voluntary movement.

Antagonists: agents that block or inhibit the working of the site or receptor on which they act. See also agonists.

Anticholinergic drugs: drugs that oppose acetylcholine, the neurotransmitter which, relative to dopamine, is increased in Parkinson's disease.

Arm swing: the ability of the arms to swing naturally and without deliberate attempt during walking.

Basal ganglia: large groups of nerve cells deep in the grey matter of the brain.

Bilateral: affecting both sides of the body; unilateral means on one side only.

Bradykinesia: slowness of movement.

Dementia: a decline in intellect, memory and the ability to make rational decisions and judgements.

Disorientation: loss of sense of time, place (where you are) and person (who you are).

Dopamine: one of a number of transmitters, made in the basal ganglia, and deficient in Parkinson's disease and some related disorders.

Dopamine agonists: drugs that drive or stimulate the working of surviving dopamine receptor cells from which dopamine is released.

Dopaminergic: dopamine forming (for example, levodopa) or dopamine stimulating, for the receptors (for example, pergolide).

Dyskinesia: abnormal movements other than tremor, which in Parkinson's disease is caused by drugs. They are often writhing, twitching or jerking movements.

Facies: the appearance of the faces often immobile or like a mask in Parkinson's disease.

Globus pallidus: one of the pairs of nerve nuclei that make up the basal ganglia.

Lewy bodies: small areas (inclusions) in nerve cells present in practically every Parkinson's disease patient. They appear, under the microscope, as pink blobs, and show a central core with a peripheral halo.

Lewy body disease: a mixture of parkinsonism with dementia in which there is a high density of Lewy bodies, not only in the deep grey matter but also in the mantle or cortex of the brain.

Mitochondria: small parts of a cell that are involved in producing energy. Mitochondrial DNA is passed from mother (not father) to children.

MPTP: methylphenyltetrahydropyridine; heroin-like drug that can cause Parkinson's disease.

Multi-system atrophy: a disorder in which there are widespread areas of shrinkage of multiple systems of nerve cells in the brain. Parkinsonism is preceded or followed by loss of blood pressure control, sweating and bladder function (autonomic dysfunction).

Neurotransmitters: the chemicals (for example, adrenaline or epinephrine, dopamine, acetylcholine) that transmit nerve impulses.

Oxidative stress: the release of oxygen compounds (toxic free radicals) by cells which act as a stress that damages cells.

Pallidotomy: the surgical destruction of the globus pallidus.

Positron emission tomography: a technique using radioactive substances to study the function of the brain.

Posture: refers to the position of the body or limbs.

Progressive supranuclear palsy: a degenerative condition with limited movements of the eyes, impaired speech and voice as well as parkinsonism.

Rigidity: stiffness, a sense of resistance to active movement.

Seborrhoea: the greasiness (resulting from secretion from seborrhoeic glands) of the skin seen in some normal people and marked in some patients with Parkinson's disease.

Stereotactic surgery: the accurate placement of a lesion by an instrument held in a rigid frame, applied to the skull, fitted with rulers, to locate the target area in three dimensions.

Substantia nigra: the black substance forming part of the basal ganglia; it is rich in dopamine cells which connect and drive other parts of the brain to achieve normal movement.

Subthalamic nucleus: one of the deeply sited pairs of nerve nuclei that make up the basal ganglia.

Transmitters: chemicals that transmit, that is, pass on, a message from one cell to the next, either stimulating or inhibiting the function concerned. It is like electricity which acts as the transmitter of sound waves in the radio.

Tremor: shaking, of the limbs or body, at rest, during posture or in movement.

Unilateral: affecting one side of the body.

Useful information

We have included the following organisations because, on preliminary investigation, they may be of use to the reader. However, we do not have first-hand experience of each organisation and so cannot guarantee the organisation's integrity. The reader must therefore exercise his or her own discretion and judgement when making further enquiries.

AbilityNet

PO Box 94
Warwickshire CV34 5WS
Information line and minicom: 0800 269545
Fax: 01926 407 425
Email: enquiries@abilitynet.org.uk
Website: www.abilitynet.org.uk

Information on specialist assistive technology to help people with any disability to use a computer. Can assess individual needs with home visits and recommend suitable equipment. Arranges training courses for employers.

Age Concern England

Astral House, 1268 London Road
London SW16 4ER
Tel: 020 8765 7200
Fax: 020 8765 7211
Helpline: 0800 009966
Email: ace@ace.org.uk
Website: www.ageconcern.org.uk

Researches into the needs of elderly people and is
involved in policy-making. Publishes many books and
has useful fact sheets on a wide range of issues from
benefits to care; provides services via local branches.

Aremco

Grove House, Lenham
Kent ME17 2PX
Tel: 01622 858 502
Fax: 01622 850 532
Email: aremco@onetel.com

Mail order company supplying information on
thousands of products including aids for people with
disabilities. For data sheets, please send an SAE.

Benefits Enquiry Line

Tel: 0800 882200
Minicom: 0800 243 355
Website: www.dwp.gov.uk
N. Ireland: 0800 220674

Government agency giving information and advice on
sickness and disability benefits for people with
disabilities and their carers.

British Association of Occupational Therapists
106–114 Borough High Street
London SE1 1LB
Tel: 020 7357 6480
Website: www.cot.org.uk

Information about all aspects of occupational therapy.
An SAE requested.

Carers UK
20–25 Glasshouse Yard
London EC1A 4JT
Tel: 020 7490 8818
Fax: 020 7490 8824
Email: info@ukcarers.org
Helpline: 0808 808 7777 (Wed, Thurs 10am–12 noon,
2–4pm)
Website: www.carersonline.org.uk

Offers information and support to all people who are
unpaid carers, looking after others with medical or
other problems.

Chartered Society of Physiotherapy
14 Bedford Row
London WC1R 4ED
Tel: 020 7306 6666
Fax: 020 7306 6611
Email: csp@csphysio.org.uk
Website: www.csp.org.uk

Information about all aspects of physiotherapy.

Chester-Care

Shelley Close, Lowmoor Business Park
Kirkby-in-Ashfield, Notts NG17 7ET
Tel: 0870 242 3234
Fax: 01623 755585
Email: homecraft@ability1.com
Website: www.homecraft-rolyan.com

Mail order company offering a wide range of items
and equipment suitable for people with disabilities.
Catalogue on request.

Citizens Advice Bureaux
(National Association of CABs)

Myddelton House, 115–123 Pentonville Road
London N1 9LZ
Tel: 020 7833 2181
Fax: 020 7833 4371
Website: www.citizensadvice.org.uk

HQ of national charity offering a wide variety of
practical, financial and legal advice. Network of local
branches throughout the UK listed in phone books and
in Yellow Pages under Counselling and Advice.

Continence Foundation

307 Hatton Square, 16 Baldwins Gardens
London EC1N 7RJ
Tel: 020 7404 6875
Fax: 020 7404 6876
Help line: 0845 345 0165 (Mon–Fri 9.30am–1pm)
Email: continence-help@dial.pipex.com
Website: www.continence-foundation.org.uk

Offers information and support for people with bladder and/or bowel problems. Has list of regional specialists. An SAE requested.

Counsel and Care

Twyman House, Bonny Street
London NW1 9PG
Tel: 020 7241 8555
Fax: 020 7267 6877
Helpline: 0845 300 7585 (Mon–Fri 10am–12noon, 2–4pm, except Wed pm)
Email: advice@counselandcare.org.uk
Website: www.counselandcare.org.uk

Information and advice on care homes, community care and housing with care.

Crossroads Caring for Carers

10 Regent Place
Rugby, Warwickshire CV21 2PN
Tel: 01788 573653
Fax: 01788 565498
Helpline: 0845 450 0350
Email: communications@crossroads.org.uk
Website: www.crossroads.org.uk

Supports and delivers high-quality services for carers and people with care needs via its local branches.
Additional helplines:
Scotland 0141 226 3793
Wales 029 2022 2282

DIAL UK
St Catherine's, Tickhill Road, Balby
Doncaster, Yorkshire DN4 8QN
Tel/minicom: 01302 310123
Fax: 01302 310404
Email: informationenquiries@dialuk.org.uk
Website: www.dialuk.org.uk

Nationwide network offering information and advice
on all aspects of disability; 130 drop-in centres run by
and for people with disabilities.

**Disabled Drivers Association (merged with
Disabled Drivers Motor Club)**
Ashwellthorpe
Norwich NR16 1EX
Tel: 0870 770 3333
Fax: 01508 488173
Email: hq@dda.org.uk
Website: www.dda.org.uk

Provides information for drivers with a disability on a
wide range of issues.

Disabled Living Foundation
380–384 Harrow Road
London W9 2HU
Tel: 020 7289 6111
Fax: 020 7266 2922
Helpline: 0845 130 9177
Textphone 020 7432 8009
Website: www.dlf.org.uk

Provides information to disabled and elderly people on all kinds of equipment in order to promote their independence and quality of life.

European Parkinson's Disease Association
4 Golding Road
Sevenoaks, Kent TN13 3NJ
Tel/Fax: 01732 457683
Email: lizzie@epda.eu.com
Website: www.epda.eu.com

Umbrella body for network of international Parkinson's disease groups, campaigning on behalf of all sufferers. Information leaflets on request. An SAE requested.

Gardening for the Disabled
c/o Julia Sebline, Hayes Farm, Hayes Lane
Peasmarsh, Kent TN31 6XR
Tel: 01424 882345
Website: www.otford.org/garden

Volunteers offer practical advice and information to help keen gardeners keep gardening despite disability or age. Offers some small grants.

Institute for Complementary Medicine
PO Box 194
London SE16 7QZ
Tel: 020 7237 5165
Fax: 020 7237 5175
Email: info@i-c-m.org.uk
Website: www.i-c-m.org.uk

Umbrella group for complementary medicine organisations. Offers informed, safe choice to public. An SAE requested.

Keep Able

3–4 Sterling Park, Pedmore Road
Brierley Hill, W, Midlands DY51 1TB
Tel: 0870 520 2122
Fax: 01384 473716
Email: homeshopping@keepable.co.uk
Website: www.keepable.co.uk

Nationwide chain of stores, advising and supplying a wide range of products for people with disabilities.

Leonard Cheshire

30 Millbank, London SW1P 4QD
Tel: 020 7802 8200
Fax: 020 7802 8250
Email: info@lc-uk.org
Website: www.leonard-cheshire.org

Offers care, support and a wide range of information for disabled people aged between 18 and 65 years in the UK and worldwide to encourage independent living. Has respite and residential homes; offers holidays and rehabilitation.

Motability Operations

City Gate House, 22 Southwark Bridge Road
London SE1 9HB
Tel: 0845 456 4566
Fax: 020 7928 1818
Website: www.motability.co.uk

Helps drivers with disabilities to access specialist cars and funding with Motability car schemes.

National Institute for Health and Clinical Excellence (NICE)

MidCity Place, 71 High Holborn
London WC1V 6NA
Tel: 020 7067 5800
Fax: 020 7067 5801
Email: nice@nice.nhs.uk
Website: www.nice.org.uk

Provides national guidance on the promotion of good health and treatment of ill-health. Patient information leaflets are available for each piece of guidance issued.

Parkinson's Disease Society (PDS)

National Office, 215 Vauxhall Bridge Road
London SW1V 1EJ
Helpline: 0808 800 0303
Tel: 020 7931 8080
Fax: 020 7233 9908
Minicom: 020 7963 9380
Email: enquiries@parkinsons.org.uk
Website: www.parkinsons.org.uk

Offers information and support via its local groups. Has nurse specialists and welfare department, and funds research into Parkinson's disease.

Prodigy Website

Sowerby Centre for Health Informatics at Newcastle
(SCHIN), Bede House, All Saints Business Centre
Newcastle on Tyne NE1 2ES
Tel: 0191 243 6100
Fax: 0191 243 6101
Email: prodigy-enquiries@schin.co.uk
Website: www.prodigy.nhs.uk/PILS/indexself.asp

A website mainly for GPs giving information for patients
listed by disease plus named self-help organisations.

PSPalsy Association (Progressive Supranuclear Palsy Association)

The Old Rectory, Wappenham
Towcester, Northants NN12 8SQ
Tel: 01327 860299
Fax: 01327 861113
Helplines: 01939 270889 (north) 01604 844825 (south)
Email: psp@pspeur.org
Website: www.pspeur.org

Offers information and support to sufferers of this rare
degenerative disease and their families.

RADAR (Royal Association for Disability and Rehabilitation)

12 City Forum, 250 City Road
London EC1V 8AF
Tel: 020 7250 3222
Fax: 020 7250 0212
Minicom: 020 7250 4119
Email: radar@radar.org.uk
Website: www.radar.org.uk

Campaigns to improve the rights and care of disabled people. Sells special key to access locked disabled toilets £3.50.

Royal College of Speech and Language Therapy

2 White Hart Yard
London SE1 1NX
Tel: 020 7378 1200
Website: www.rcslt.org

Information about all aspects of speech and language therapy.

Thrive

The Geoffrey Udall Centre, Beech Hill
Reading, Berks RG7 2AT
Tel: 0118 988 5688
Fax: 0118 988 5677
Helpline for blind gardeners: 0118 988 6668
Website: www.thrive.org.uk

Has several projects nationally offering opportunities to people with disabilities to improve their skills and gain qualifications in gardening and horticulture

Tourism for All (previously Holiday Care)

c/o Vitalise, Shap Road Industrial Estate, Shap Road
Kendal, Cumbria LA9 6NZ
Tel: 0845 124 9974
Fax: 0845 124 9972
Helpline: 0845 124 9971
Email: info@tourismforall.org.uk
Website: www.tourismforall.org.uk

Provides information to people with disabilities on transport, holiday accommodation, activity holidays and respite care establishments in the UK and abroad. See Vitalise below.

Tripscope

The Vassal Centre, Gill Avenue
Bristol BS16 2QQ
Tel: 0845 758 5641
Fax: 0117 939 7736
Email: enquiries@tripscope.org.uk
Website: www.tripscope.org.uk

Provides comprehensive information for elderly and disabled people on all aspects of travelling, within the UK and abroad.

Vitalise (previously Winged Fellowship Trust)

12 City Forum, 250 City Road
London EC1V 8AF
Tel: 0845 345 1972
Fax: 0845 345 1978
Email: info@vitalise.org.uk
Website: www.vitalise.org.uk

Offers holidays at their own centres and overseas and respite care for people with severe disabilities by providing voluntary carers. Also arranges holidays for people with Alzheimer's disease/dementia and their carers.

Websites

www.bbc.co.uk/health
Information on health matters.

The internet as a source of further information

After reading this book, you may feel that you would like further information on the subject. The internet is of course an excellent place to look and there are many websites with useful information about medical disorders, related charities and support groups.

For those who do not have a computer at home some bars and cafes offer facilities for accessing the internet. These are listed in the *Yellow Pages* under 'Internet Bars and Cafes' and 'Internet Providers'. Your local library offers a similar facility and has staff to help you find the information that you need.

It should always be remembered, however, that the internet is unregulated and anyone is free to set up a website and add information to it. Many websites offer impartial advice and information that has been compiled and checked by qualified medical professionals. Some, on the other hand, are run by commercial organisations with the purpose of promoting their own products. Others still are run by pressure groups, some of which will provide carefully assessed and accurate information whereas others may be suggesting medications or treatments that are not supported by the medical and scientific community.

Unless you know the address of the website you want to visit – for example, www.familydoctor.co.uk – you may find the following guidelines useful when searching the internet for information.

Search engines and other searchable sites

Google (www.google.co.uk) is the most popular search engine used in the UK, followed by Yahoo! (http://uk.

yahoo.com) and MSN (www.msn.co.uk). Also popular
are the search engines provided by Internet Service
Providers such as Tiscali and other sites such as the
BBC site (www.bbc.co.uk).

In addition to the search engines that index the
whole web, there are also medical sites with search
facilities, which act almost like mini-search engines, but
cover only medical topics or even a particular area of
medicine. Again, it is wise to look at who is responsible
for compiling the information offered to ensure that it
is impartial and medically accurate. The NHS Direct site
(www.nhsdirect.nhs.uk) is an example of a searchable
medical site.

Links to many British medical charities can be found
at the Association of Medical Research Charities'
website (www.amrc.org.uk) and at Charity Choice
(www.charitychoice.co.uk).

Search phrases

Be specific when entering a search phrase. Searching
for information on 'cancer' will return results for many
different types of cancer as well as on cancer in
general. You may even find sites offering astrological
information. More useful results will be returned by
using search phrases such as 'lung cancer' and
'treatments for lung cancer'. Both Google and Yahoo!
offer an advanced search option that includes the
ability to search for the exact phrase; enclosing the
search phrase in quotes, that is, 'treatments for lung
cancer', will have the same effect. Limiting a search to
an exact phrase reduces the number of results returned
but it is best to refine a search to an exact match only
if you are not getting useful results with a normal
search. Adding 'UK' to your search term will bring up

mainly British sites, so a good phrase might be 'lung cancer' UK (don't include UK within the quotes).

Always remember the internet is international and unregulated. It holds a wealth of valuable information but individual sites may be biased, out of date or just plain wrong. Family Doctor Publications accepts no responsibility for the content of links published in this series.

Index

Your pages

We have included the following pages because they may help you manage your illness or condition and its treatment.

Before an appointment with a health professional, it can be useful to write down a short list of questions of things that you do not understand, so that you can make sure that you do not forget anything.

Some of the sections may not be relevant to your circumstances.

We are always pleased to receive constructive criticism or suggestions about how to improve the books. You can contact us at:

Email: familydoctor@btinternet.com
Letter: Family Doctor Publications
         PO Box 4664
         Poole
         BH15 1NN

Thank you

Health-care contact details

Name:

Job title:

Place of work:

Tel:

Name:

Job title:

Place of work:

Tel:

Name:

Job title:

Place of work:

Tel:

Name:

Job title:

Place of work:

Tel:

Significant past health events – illnesses/ operations/investigations/treatments

Event	Month	Year	Age (at time)

Appointments for health care

Name:

Place:

Date:

Time:

Tel:

Name:

Place:

Date:

Time:

Tel:

Name:

Place:

Date:

Time:

Tel:

Name:

Place:

Date:

Time:

Tel:

Appointments for health care

Name:

Place:

Date:

Time:

Tel:

Name:

Place:

Date:

Time:

Tel:

Name:

Place:

Date:

Time:

Tel:

Name:

Place:

Date:

Time:

Tel:

Current medication(s) prescribed by your doctor

Medicine name:

Purpose:

Frequency & dose:

Start date:

End date:

Medicine name:

Purpose:

Frequency & dose:

Start date:

End date:

Medicine name:

Purpose:

Frequency & dose:

Start date:

End date:

Medicine name:

Purpose:

Frequency & dose:

Start date:

End date:

Other medicines/supplements you are taking, not prescribed by your doctor

Medicine/treatment:

Purpose:

Frequency & dose:

Start date:

End date:

Medicine/treatment:

Purpose:

Frequency & dose:

Start date:

End date:

Medicine/treatment:

Purpose:

Frequency & dose:

Start date:

End date:

Medicine/treatment:

Purpose:

Frequency & dose:

Start date:

End date:

Questions to ask at appointments
(Note: do bear in mind that doctors work under great time pressure, so long lists may not be helpful for either of you)

Questions to ask at appointments
(Note: do bear in mind that doctors work under great time pressure, so long lists may not be helpful for either of you)

Notes